9 Steps for Reversing or Preventing Cancer

and Other Diseases

Learn to Heal From Within

9 Steps for Reversing or Preventing Cancer

and Other Diseases

Learn to Heal From Within

Shivani Goodman, Ed.D.

Foreword by Jack Canfield

Introduction by O. Carl Simonton, M.D.

New Page Books
A division of The Career Press, Inc.
Franklin Lakes, NJ

9 STEPS FOR REVERSING OR PREVENTING CANCER AND OTHER DISEASES
EDITED AND TYPESET BY NANCY J. HAJESKI
Cover design by Foster & Foster, Inc.
Printed in the U.S.A. by Book-mart Press

Excerpts from the self-help guide to O. Carl Simonton's
Getting Well program appear with permission.

To order this title, please call toll-free 1-800-CAREER-1 (NJ and Canada: 201-848-0310) to order using VISA or MasterCard, or for further information on books from Career Press.

 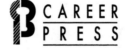

The Career Press, Inc., 3 Tice Road, PO Box 687,
Franklin Lakes, NJ 07417
www.careerpress.com
www.newpagebooks.com

Library of Congress Cataloging-in-Publication Data

Goodman, Shivani.
    9 steps for reversing or preventing cancer and other diseases : learn to heal fromnwithin / by Shivani Goodman ; foreword by Jack Canfield ; introduction by O. Carl Simonton.
        p. cm.
    Includes index.
    ISBN 1-56414-749-5 (pbk.)
        1. Mental healing. 2. Medicine, Psychosomatic. 3. Psychoneuroimmunology. I. Title:Nine steps for reversing or preventing cancer and other diseases. II. Title.

RZ400.G687 2004
616.08--dc22

                                                                                        2004040252

Dedication

To my son, Steven—
You have been the best son a mother can wish for.
You are a beacon of light and my inspiration.

To your honesty and openness,
dear students and clients worldwide—you are my teachers.

I also dedicate this book to you, dear reader,
to own and be your full potential.

Acknowledgments

I am eternally grateful to O. Carl Simonton, M.D., for being a pioneer in the mind/body field and for helping me in my journey with cancer. He taught me the health value of a belief, the healing power of healthy decisions, and to see my cancer as a message of love. What I learned from him inspired me to go on and develop my own program.

I am eternally grateful to Babaji Maha Avatar Haidakhandi for guiding me on the spiritual path: that every human being be benefited and liberated.

I am eternally grateful to you, Hanne Strong, for your encouragement to heal myself.

I am grateful to John, my ex-husband, for sharing 32 years of my life.

I am grateful to Sharon Rose for creating the Healing Circles. And I am grateful for her superb ability to take my work and create a book.

I thank Soma Krishna for teaching me the Tibetan healing exercise, which helped me so much in my own healing.

I thank Bud Feder, Ph.D., for teaching me Gestalt therapy.

I thank Les Fehmi, Ph.D., director of the Biofeedback Institute in Princeton, N.J., for teaching me the pain relief exercise.

I thank Dolores Krieger for her research and work in Therapeutic Touch and Master Mantak Chia for teaching me the healing energy circuit exercise.

I also thank Deepak Chopra, M.D.; Bernie Siegel, M.D.; Dean Ornish, M.D.; Gerald Jampolsky, M.D.; Arnold Lazarus, Ph.D.; Richard Alpert, Ph.D.; Wayne Dyer, Ph.D.; Laura Perls, Ph.D.; Richard Erskine, Ph.D.; Chris Gilbert, Ph.D.; Milton Klein, Ph.D.; Tim O'Connel, Ph.D.; Marianne Williamson; Neale Donald Walsh; Louise Hay; Stephen Covey; Thomas Moore; David Whyte;

Tirza Moussaieff, M.A.; Barbara Rosenbaum, Ph.D.; Elaine Braff, M.A.; Sharon Fraquamont, Ph.D.; Dr. Laurie Eaton; Dr. Ilchi Lee; Howard Wills; Shri Chinmoy; Dr. Zengo Yaul; and R. Ibrahim Jaffe, M.D. for all that they have taught me.

I am deeply grateful to my parents, Remo and Leah, who taught me to be courageous...and to my eleven magnificent brothers and sisters—I thank you for *being* in my life!

—S.G.

Disclaimer

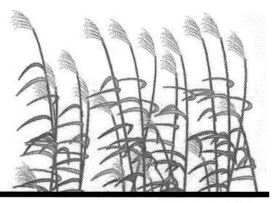

The 9-Steps Program to Reverse or Prevent Cancer and Other Diseases is not meant to replace medical advice or treatment.* Ask the healers and healthcare professionals who specialize in your problem area to guide you.

This book is based on my experience and observations made while learning how to reverse my own cancer and other diseases, as well as working with thousands of clients and workshop participants suffering from disease. These are the tools that have helped so many all over the world.

I don't heal other people. I teach people how to go to the cause of disease and heal themselves from within. Changes happen from the inside out. Unless you heal the underlying cause, disease may come back again. I give you the tools so you can do it yourself using the wisdom that is within you. Use this book as a guide to help you find your own inner wisdom and what feels right for you. Take what works and disregard the rest.

The names of my clients have been changed except where permission has been given to reveal true identities.

My goal in writing this book is to help ease pain, suffering, and sickness, thereby bringing more balance and well-being to this world. May this book be an adventure into new ways of thinking, living, and healing.

The purpose of this book is to educate, and it is sold with the understanding that the author and publisher shall have neither liability nor responsibility for any injury caused or alleged to be caused directly or indirectly by the information or advice contained in this book.

Contents

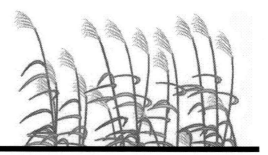

Foreword

I met Shivani Goodman at the Maui Writers Conference where I teach each year. I had just spotted Shivani's first book, *Lessons From the Master: One Woman's Journey to Self-Healing*, in the hands of a good friend of mine and was inquiring where I could get a copy when, at that very moment, Shivani passed by and my friend invited her to join us.

Shivani asked me if I would be interested in experiencing a five-minute exercise that had recently helped a physician heal his colon cancer within one week.

"Absolutely," I responded, always being open to experiencing something new that might be of use to others. "Let's meet in 10 minutes," I added.

As I was walking to meet Shivani, I spontaneously pointed to two other people I knew and said, "You and you, come with me." There were about eight people sitting together on the far corner of the patio as Shivani guided us though her exercise. When I opened my eyes at the end of the five-minute experience, I was feeling total bliss.

"The Five-Minute Cure," I said to Shivani, "that's what I'd call it."

Then I learned that what Dr. Goodman is up to is in alignment with my deepest values of empowering ordinary people to lead extraordinary lives. She has devoted her life to preventing pain, sickness, and suffering.

As a former psychologist with 25 years of hands-on experience helping thousands of people worldwide, Shivani discovered in 1992 that she had breast cancer. At first she thought it was a joke. Here she had been teaching the techniques of self-healing only to find herself in a condition similar to that of her patients and clients.

She now had to make a decision. Go the conventional route of surgery, chemotherapy, and radiation or try her own method of self-healing. What followed was a roller-coaster ride from doubt to conviction, from deep sadness to great joy, which she so eloquently expresses in this book.

It was this defining moment in her life that gave her deep insights into herself and the mind/body connection. Realizing the gift that she received through her new insights, she used her concept to forge a program and foundation of self-healing that she has been teaching in classes and seminars for the past several years. And her students can attest to the miracles they have experienced as they realized the power of one's own mind to heal.

In this excellent book, Dr. Goodman shows how you can take command of your own life and heal yourself instead of turning over the responsibility to a doctor or a third party.

Dr. Goodman takes you through the process of visualization, ancient self-healing technology, and identifies the self-toxic attitudes that create the illness or pain in the first place.

Unlike many books on healing, Dr. Goodman's cites a step-by-step method that has created wonderful results—so much so that she has devoted her life to teaching these methods to others in seminars and workshops.

My hat's off to a woman who continues to do so much good for those willing to explore the proven and often subtle methods she teaches. For it is within these pages that her work will expand, and the good that she has already done will be magnified many-fold. I am proud to know this fine teacher and the work that she has done. And I am happy that you, too, now get to reap the benefits of her commitment to health and healing.

—Jack Canfield
    Cocreator of the *Chicken Soup for the Soul* series;
    Coauthor of *Chicken Soup for the Healthy Soul*

Introduction

For the past 32 years, I have studied the powerful connection between the mind and healing.

As a medical doctor and radiation oncologist, I know well the current methods that cancer treatment requires. However, 32 years ago, I elected to address the minds and emotions of my patients in addition to traditional medicine and coauthored one of the first books on the mind/body connection titled, *Getting Well Again*.

The book was well received and eventually was translated into 32 languages and became a best-seller. Since that time, I have advocated the power of the mind/body connection to heal and to effect dramatic transformations in the lives of those who are suffering pain and sickness. I have developed standardized counseling processes and standardized training of counselors internationally.

Dr. Goodman's book is a do-it-yourself manual for healing. A unique feature of this book is the ability of the author to teach people how to go within and heal themselves. Goodman says that she doesn't heal others, she shows people how to be their own therapist—how to connect with the doctor within and find answers to solve any problem in life, be it cancer, a relationship crisis, or a financial challenge.

9 Steps for Reversing or Preventing Cancer and Other Diseases is also a guide to using the intelligence of the body to heal itself. The book features ancient healing-guided imagery and simple exercises from the latest research on mind/body medicine. The processes provide guidance on how to change toxic self-sabotaging attitudes and how to empower the individual to know that one has the ability to be healthy and feel joy.

9 Steps for Reversing or Preventing Cancer and Other Diseases

From time to time certain books appear that help shift the consciousness of humanity to a new level of understanding and healing. These books that show you how to feel joy, love, and peace and increase your health and the quality of life are a rare gift to us. I consider *9 Steps for Reversing or Preventing Cancer and Other Diseases* to be such a gift. The intention of this work is apparent: to decrease sickness, pain, and suffering from people's lives. I believe that the guidance is simple and very clear in doing just that. The processes about self-healing from a psychologist's experience with her own advanced cancer enhanced her ability to help others. See for yourself as you read this excellent guide to good health. Dr. Goodman is on a path that I personally feel is the medicine of the future.

Many spiritual disciplines teach the concept that illness is a blessing. It is a signal that something we are doing is fundamentally interfering with our harmonious nature. The purpose of the illness is to increase our awareness of the problem so we can correct the problem and grow through the process of self-healing. It is also communicated clearly that no guilt or self-blame is indicated, as these emotions would simply cause more suffering and more illness.

To me, Dr. Goodman's book helps guide us through this process.

—O. Carl Simonton, M.D.
author of *Getting Well Again*

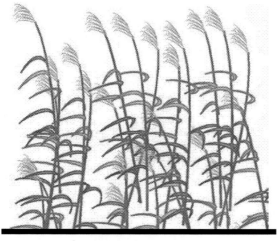

Part 1

Finding the Cause of
Cancer and Other Diseases

Chapter 1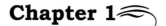

Using the Mind/Body Connection to Get to the Cause

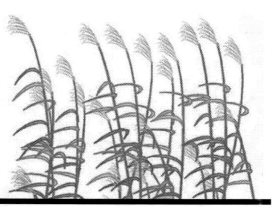

"My sister had breast cancer nearly 10 years ago, and now she has been diagnosed with terminal bone cancer," Jack told me over the phone. "Angela's doctors said there is nothing they can do to help her—not even surgery or chemotherapy will stop the cancer."

I first met Jack at a United Nations conference in Istanbul, and we'd kept in touch over the years. I now offered to teach Angela my program of self-healing exercises. The next day, they both flew from Paris to meet with me.

Angela was pale as a ghost and hunched over. She couldn't walk without a cane. Her eyes bulged in terror. She was consumed with the fear of dying—and with another fear: Her 19-year-old daughter was very attached to her mother, and she'd told Angela she could not live without her.

While we worked through the Daily Healing Routine, Angela remembered a number of childhood experiences in which she'd felt abandoned, unwanted, and rejected by her parents. At 7, she was sent to boarding school when her parents divorced. She thought she'd been sent away because she did something wrong.

"I believed that I was stupid, ugly, and unlovable," Angela said. "The words, 'Get away from me, you are not wanted,' suddenly bubbled up from my memory. I remembered fearing my father—who hit me—and my stepmother—who criticized me. I learned to feel afraid of everybody I knew. I became invisible and quiet, as if I didn't exist. I was very timid, always trying to do and say the right thing so people wouldn't get angry with me. Since I was yelled at constantly, I decided that I was inferior, a failure. As these memories came up, I felt deep pain in my heart and spine.

"When I practiced the five-minute self-healing exercise, it felt so good to fill my pain with love. As I continued the exercises, I imagined myself talking to my inner self, and she slowly began to feel better. I saw her smiling, laughing, then dancing with joy and running out to play with her friends, feeling happy and having fun.

"I then realized that I was still feeling all these same negative emotions in my life now. As I became aware of that, an image of a wise older woman appeared in my mind. She was radiantly beautiful, shining with joy and health. Intuitively I knew that this was me in the future, looking youthful. I heard her say to me the same words I had said to the little girl. She showed me my future as exciting and fulfilling.

"I realized then that my cancer and my difficulties in life were covering up the real issue of being disconnected from my true essence of love and joy. I also realized that my feelings of shame and lack of self-love were destroying my body.

"As this new awareness settled in, a soft, gentle sensation of love bubbled up in my heart. I felt like I was coming home to my real self. I knew this love was what was going to heal me. For the first time I could smell the flowers in the room. I opened my eyes feeling elated, knowing that I will heal."

When Angela practiced the exercise, "creating bliss and finding your passion," an image appeared in her mind's eye of her enjoying time with her future grandchildren. She later wrote to me, "Within two days of practicing your method, my pain became a lot less severe, and I started walking without my cane. I totally forgot that I couldn't walk without it."

A neighbor of mine who met Angela on the elevator asked me, "What happened? She looked like death when I saw her two days ago. Now she is a new person, laughing and smiling, and her face is rosy and radiant. I find it hard to believe it's the same woman."

After they returned home, Angela's brother, who was an alcoholic and had attended some of our sessions, called to say, "Not only did my sister heal, *I* healed too. I am no longer experiencing emotional and mental pain. I have stopped drinking. I am very grateful."

A year later, Angela wrote, "The tumor on my ribcage has shrunk dramatically, and my doctors are telling me that I am no longer terminal; they can now operate on me. I refused their recommendation and continue working on my self-healing. I feel that your program saved my life. I am feeling great."

Angela later told me that she had continued to do the exercises, and now she is pain-free—physically as well as emotionally—and in good health. She joyfully told me that she was babysitting for her newly arrived first grandchild.

Two months later, Angela called to tell me that she went in for a checkup, and her blood test was normal. Her doctor told her she is in remission, and he doesn't need to see her for another six months. She was amazed that exactly five years ago the doctors had told her that she was terminal.

Unfortunately, few people have learned the self-healing techniques that saved Angela's life. One in every four deaths in America is from cancer, and half of all Americans living today, or *more than 92 million* people, will get cancer during their lifetime. *Forty percent of those diagnosed with cancer this year will not be alive in five years.* More children under age 15 die from cancer than any other disease. And the death rate continues to rise as cancer is predicted to soon replace heart disease as the number-one killer. In addition, millions are suffering from other diseases that limit or interrupt the quality of life.

Not only are the current treatments not working, they cost a small fortune, which threatens the financial security of families across the country. The National Cancer Institute estimates that cancer costs Americans $60 billion a year in medical bills. Looking at other diseases, such as heart disease, just one heart bypass operation can cost as much as $50,000. Sadly, many patients have had this procedure done three times.

What I have learned from mind/body medicine is that surgery and drugs only remove the symptoms of disease, not the cause. Unless the cause is healed, diseases such as heart disease and cancer will reoccur. Experience has shown me that our self-sabotaging attitudes are like poison to the body, weakening and eventually disabling our immune systems, creating disease. Changing these toxic attitudes to healing decisions enables the body to heal itself. Symptoms are messages from the body that our toxic attitudes are having a detrimental effect on the body.

My own triumph over cancer and my work with those who challenge disease all around the world have taught me that cancer and other diseases are the result of denying our inherent goodness and worthiness, and identifying with not being good or worthy enough. We then become filled with fear and doubt—rather than the love and joy of our true self—and the body begins to break down.

This book details the program that reversed my cancer and that has helped so many of my clients and workshop participants worldwide do the same. You will be shown how to find the psychological and spiritual blocks that stop the body's flow of life force, which ultimately cause disease, and you will be shown how to dissolve these blocks so the body can heal itself.

You will discover how you denied your needs when you made decisions against yourself. And you will be shown how to reconnect with your goodness and find your heart's bliss and passion for life that naturally bring you joy and healing. This program will show you how to heal yourself on all levels—physically, emotionally, mentally, and spiritually. Finally, you will be shown how to create a supportive healing environment that will reinforce your new healthy thinking and attitudes while you are healing.

Mind/Body Medicine and Psychoneuroimmunology

Because surgery and chemotherapy had not stopped my cancer from recurring, I knew I had to look elsewhere. On my journey back to health, I tried many different alternative therapies and visited many healers. Some were helpful up to a point, others did nothing for me, some were a waste of time and money, some made me worse, and some endangered my health. I tried special diets, detoxing my body, and even saw a Shaman. But none of these things worked for me. I couldn't bear eating unsatisfying food for the rest of my life. Enjoying tasty food has always been a source of pleasure that I didn't want to give up. What did appeal to me was the emerging field of mind/body medicine. As a psychologist, I understood how the mind affects the body.

In 1984 I founded and directed the Biofeedback, Psychology, and Stress Management Center in Livingston, N.J. I had a large private practice and helped thousands of people solve a variety of problems from emotional to physical disorders. I became known for my expertise in reversing psychosomatic disorders using Gestalt therapy, biofeedback and self hypnosis. The beneficial combination of these modalities led me to develop a program that helped alleviate many physiological disorders, such as hypertension, ulcers, arthritis, rheumatism, headaches, and back pain. All kinds of aches and pains were successfully treated. I also dealt with anxiety, depression, phobias, relationship problems, and other psychological disorders on a daily basis. This combination of modalities was helpful in all the cases I dealt with.

My research into biofeedback showed me how the mind affects the body. In addition, numerous validated research findings confirmed the ability to reverse physiological disorders with the mind. I understood that *there is a physiological response in every cell of the body to every thought we think.*

When cancer appeared in my life, I started exploring the possibility that the mind/body connection theories would also apply to cancer. I studied extensively, researching articles and participating in many programs and seminars. I first learned about the field of scientific research called psychoneuroimmunology, or PNI, from O. Carl Simonton, M.D., a pioneer in mind/body medicine, when I attended his five-day seminar in Los Angeles.

Broken down into its parts, psychoneuroimmunology means thoughts (psycho) affect the nervous system (neuro) and then affect the immune system (immunology). Dr. Simonton introduced validated research findings that showed how negative thoughts, which produce emotional stress (in our nervous system), affect our immune systems.

The *Getting Well Audio Program Guidebook* by Simonton states on page 17:

> "The immune system—the body's natural defense—is designed to contain or destroy any cancerous cells, which current medical thinking suggests we all have in our bodies from time to time. Suppression of the immune system, however, can result in cancerous growth. Emotional stress...produces a suppression of the immune system, which leaves the body susceptible to the development of cancer."

Creating an Environment for Disease to Grow

Because our bodies have the innate ability to heal and repair from the effects of stress, injury, and disease, what creates the environment for disease to develop? PNI research indicates that *the thoughts, attitudes, beliefs, and images we hold in our mind affect our emotions and our nervous and immune systems.* Our emotional and mental states have the potential to weaken or activate the immune system against disease.

The *Getting Well Audio Program Guidebook* continues on page 8:

"The important point here is that something is happening in the person who contracts the cancer to create susceptibility....What lapse in the body's defenses allows these cells to reproduce into a life-threatening tumor at this time? What inhibits the body's immune system from performing the function that it has performed successfully for many years?

"The answers to these questions bring us back to emotional and mental factors in health and illness. The same factors that may determine why one patient lives and another with the identical diagnosis and treatment dies also influence why one person contracts a disease and another does not."

For example, PNI research shows that everyone who smokes doesn't get cancer. The *Getting Well Audio Program Guidebook* states:

"...when exposed to known cancer-producing substances, most people still remain healthy...if all it took to get cancer was exposure to nicotine and tars, then all heavy smokers would contract the disease. *Yet most heavy smokers do not get lung cancer.* [italics added by author]

"...there are substantially different incidence rates for cancer among patients with different kinds of mental and emotional problems. These clues point to significant connections between emotional states and illness."

What Toxic Attitudes Do to the Body

The latest research in PNI shows that *our negative thoughts and emotions slowly destroy our immune system until disease occurs.* These negative thoughts and emotions solidify into attitudes that are toxic to the body and make us sick. Strong sarcastic, skeptical, pessimistic attitudes create energy blockages that stop the flow of vital life-force energy (hormones, chemicals, and nutrients that are usually carried to all parts of the body) depleting the immune system until disease starts. If these destructive attitudes are not changed, the discomfort grows and the sickness gets worse, eventually killing us.

From my experience working with cancer and other disease patients all over the world using the program presented in Part II of this book, I have determined that it is our psychological and spiritual blocks that prevent us from radiant health. Having also studied numerous ancient healing traditions for more than 30 years, I have learned that psychological issues that have not been resolved create internal tension. That tension blocks the flow of the life-force in the body/mind systems. These blockages are the reason for the diseases that develop in the physical body.

Dr. Margo de Kooker, a medical doctor specializing in the field of behavioral medicine, states in "An Overview of Psychoneuroimmunology," her January 1999 article for *Rennaissance Magazine*:

> "What the field of PNI tells us is that every part of our immune system is connected to the brain in some way....The immune system...is sensitive to...the chemicals secreted in the brain in response to our mental-emotional processing (moods and feelings).

> "PNI research helps us understand the interactions between mental and emotional states, immune system functioning, and ultimately health. *In healthcare today we have passed from the surgical revolution through the chemical revolution and have entered into the behavioral revolution.* [Italics added by author]

> "In the real world, what the field of PNI proves is that what happens in our minds at the level of our perception (and our emotional reaction to that perception) can have real effects on our immune systems. This concept is not new at all, and ancient wisdom has always encouraged us to focus on maintaining a 'healthy' mind in order to maintain a healthy body. It is only now that we are able to prove and understand the connections.

> "...lingering unresolved emotions and inflexible ways of coping can become the source of chronic low-grade stress, which can undermine immune system functioning....Given the right genetics, a weakened physical condition, or an existing illness, and you may be sitting on a time bomb."

My experience is that unresolved emotions and toxic attitudes create an internal conflict, which puts an incredible stress on the systems of the body and results in the breakdown of the immune system. Harmful or unresolved emotion can take many forms. For example, every time we worry, doubt, fear, lack, hate, judge, or resent someone or something, it literally stops the body's natural healing and rejuvenation process. First, the adrenals become stressed, then the nervous system, and finally the hormones. This continual interruption of the rhythm of the body's natural healing process—like a stop and start activity—creates a war within the body. The body starts to break down and attack itself. And the process known as disease begins.

Unresolved emotions are the result of emotional experiences from the past that you are holding onto and have never released. For example, remember the times in your life you felt betrayed, abused, taken advantage of, treated unfairly, cheated, lied to, talked about negatively, made fun of (especially in childhood), treated disrespectfully, picked on, made to feel inferior or worthless, criticized, or hurt in other ways.

These emotions are stored in the body until you have an emotional tornado lurking inside, unexpressed and repressed. And eventually they begin destroying you inside. You don't know it until you start feeling physical discomfort, such as headaches, back pain, and other aches and pains. If you don't pay attention and find ways to release the emotional blockage, the symptoms intensify and are first diagnosed as hypertension, ulcers, migraines, and the like.

Taking drugs to alleviate the symptoms is like putting a Band-Aid on a deep wound. These symptoms need to be healed at the core. The psychological cause needs to be identified and healed. Taking drugs can complicate things further. You walk around feeling emotionally unhappy for 30 or 40 years, unaware that what's probably causing that unhappiness are layers of buried anger toward another person or, more likely, many people. Then you get cancer or another disease, and you take more medication and poisons that weaken your system further. Although certain drugs do give temporary relief of some symptoms, they are not addressing the cause of your disease, which continues to grow inside.

Traditional medicine has taught us to look for the cause and cure outside of ourselves, instead of inside where the cause is waiting to be resolved so that the body can resume its normal healing process. Drugs and surgery are only temporary measures to try to alleviate the symptoms. However, drugs, surgery, changing your diet, taking vitamins, detoxing your body, and exercising will not make the disease go away unless you are also healing your emotions.

The great healer is to release the emotional pain and to get it out of your body.

Until you release the emotional pain, the body lives in a constant state of emotional stress and continues to deteriorate. And you may not even know it because you have been living that way for so many years. You don't recognize that you are stressed and filled with anguish until your body becomes diseased. Sickness is the body's way of trying to get rid of stress. When you carry long-term stress, you are "living in the past." Whatever emotional traumas you have been experiencing for years manifest in the body as disease, especially in the area of weakness and according to the thoughts you hold. If you continue to think in terms of the past and carry your unresolved emotional experiences with you, you will collapse the body.

Disease as a Solution

There is an additional point to consider. When life's problems seem insurmountable, cancer and other life-threatening illnesses can be viewed on a subconscious level as a solution.

The *Getting Well Audio Program Guidebook* states on page 16:

> "There is some considerable evidence that stress predisposes people to illness, including cancer. Research has shown that it is possible to predict major illness based on the number of stresses in people's lives in the months preceding the onset of illness. Our clinical observations confirm this clustering of major stresses in our patients' lives, but they also suggest that the effect of these stresses is even greater if they threaten some role or relationship that is central to the individual's identity or if they pose a problem or situation from which there is apparently no escape. Moreover, our studies and others suggest that these critical stresses are likely to have occurred six to 18 months prior to diagnosis of the disease.

> "...it is not just stress, but the way of reacting to stress that makes a difference in the susceptibility to disease. We have all learned rules about who we are and how we are to act, which provide the limits within which we cope with stresses. In some cases, these rules limit a person's ability to cope with stress to the point that the stresses seem to pose unsolvable problems. The result can be depression, despair, hopelessness, and helplessness—*all feelings that have been reported to precede cancer*. [Italics added by author] Because

29

of these feelings, at either a conscious or unconscious level, serious illness and/or death become acceptable as potential solutions."

Looking back to when I got cancer, this makes perfect sense. I was often feeling depressed and hopeless about having to spend the rest of my life in a stressful situation that was making me deeply unhappy. I would shut these thoughts and feelings out of my mind and dismiss them as silly. Cancer ended up being a solution to a problem that with my toxic thinking, I couldn't see any way of escaping.

What Causes the Recurrence of Cancer and Disease?

PNI allowed me to make the connection between the subconscious psychological cause and the manifestation of my cancer. In my private practice with clients, I had been researching the importance of the emotional and mental cause, which, if not resolved, will allow the cancer to reappear, sometimes somewhere else in the body as it had with me. Because my cancer kept recurring, I was aware that I had never addressed and healed the root cause.

When we get sick, the tendency is to take drugs, have surgery, or follow other recommendations made by our medical professionals. From my experience this is like putting Vaseline on a broken limb. It is true that sometimes the symptoms disappear. But what happens is that either new symptoms appear or the next attack is more vicious than the previous one, until the cause that created the sickness in the first place is resolved. Finding the emotional and mental cause is the key.

I had cancer three times before I was able to discover the toxic attitudes that caused my cancer and remove them one at a time. The first few toxic attitudes were about me being out of balance in my life—I was overworked and overstressed, seeing an average of more than 60 clients every week.

I grew up in war-torn Israel and at an early age experienced my brother being killed in the war. Later, my sister died in a terrorist attack. I decided that I wanted to help relieve all the pain and suffering and show people how to live in joy. This led me to choose the path of psychology. I eventually came to this country with my husband and got my doctorate at Columbia University. I continued to study with the great teachers of healing, including spending six years with a master healer in the foothills of the Himalayas. I wanted to learn everything I could.

I had been teaching self-healing for more than 20 years. I loved my chosen field, but I could not stop working. I was going seven days a week, nonstop. I remember having between 40 and 60 private sessions and about five group therapy sessions—*all within one week*. On top of that, I took care of cooking for my family, as well as doing laundry, bookkeeping, paperwork, reports, and on and on. I was a workaholic and did not know it.

Cancer forced me to take time out for myself. I remember feeling guilty if I snuck a few minutes to lie down and rest. I am aware that there are people who have so much energy that they work even harder than I did, yet they don't get sick. However, my toxic attitudes of guilt and lack of self worth weakened my immune system, and my body started to break down. And because of those negative attitudes, I neglected to pay attention to the small signs, the aches and pains in my upper back.

It did not occur to me to make changes in my life. It was not clear to me that my self-sabotaging attitudes and work schedule were the cause of my sickness; just as I often find that the most obvious cause is not clear to my clients and students. After my first reoccurrence, I kept asking myself, "What is the message of my cancer?" I got many responses and started acting accordingly. I began traveling to fulfill my heart's longings to be in Israel and Colorado, where many supportive friends and family members lived.

However, it wasn't until the third reoccurrence, after I embarked on a program of self-healing, that I discovered the deepest toxic attitude that was the root cause of my cancer. I would often ask myself during my daily routine of relaxation and self healing, "Why me and why my breasts?"

I discovered many minor causes, but the most critical one was revealed to me when I allowed myself to delve deeply into the pain in my upper spine near my heart. I breathed and relaxed into that area, as I have been teaching my students to do for many years. I started crying with the pain, exaggerating it, feeling it, expanding it until it became worse.

A scene from my childhood appeared in my mind's eye—one that had imprinted deep pain into my psyche about being a woman. In the Jewish tradition, men are required to pray certain prayers in the morning. One prayer that my father would say out loud every day is: "Thank you, God, for not making me a slave. Thank you, God, for not making me a woman."

I remember experiencing a deep depression about my bad luck of having been born a female.

Recalling this scene from my childhood, I was suddenly able to make sense of it all. My breasts are my symbol of femininity. Subconsciously, I was rejecting being a woman, rejecting the notion that I deserved to be alive.

When I mentioned this discovery to some religious family members and friends, they told me that I'd misunderstood the meaning of the prayer. "The reason men say that prayer is to thank God that they were made men because they couldn't handle the pain of childbirth. Women are stronger, and they are able to handle it," they said. It was also explained to me that men are required to perform good deeds, and women are not, so this is the way the men express their gratitude in this prayer.

I recommended that any little girls who would hear the prayer be told that the reason men say this prayer is to honor women's strength; they needed to understand that it was wonderful to be a woman.

Then I remembered that my grandmother died from breast cancer. I realized that this feeling of being inferior as a woman must have been an issue in my family for generations. Looking at men and women in society, I think it is a worldwide issue. The attitude of women being inferior to men has been prevalent in most cultures for centuries. It is a deeply rooted inherited toxic decision and could be the cause behind the current epidemic of breast cancer. Every year 40,000 women die from breast cancer in the United States alone. These subconscious attitudes need to be addressed, understood, integrated, and converted to feelings of well-being if women are to be happy, healthy, productive beings.

Our toxic attitudes are what break down the immune system and make us sick. The effect my toxic attitudes had on my body was recurring cancer and feelings of discomfort about myself. I wanted to be different. I wanted to be strong and good enough. However, my deeply ingrained attitudes gave me much physical pain. Attitudes such as: "I am not good enough as I am; I must be better. If I were smarter, richer, more attractive, and more successful, maybe then I would be acceptable. I am not lovable the way I am, therefore, I can't love and accept myself as I am. Being a woman makes me not worthwhile."

Once I was able to identify the core self-sabotaging attitudes I had about myself, I was able to change them into healing attitudes that healed my psyche and created radiant health.

Reversing the Cycle to Achieve Recovery and Prevention

Our emotional and mental states have the potential to weaken or activate the immune system against disease. The good news is that attitudes can be changed. They can be changed by the mere decision to be open to experimenting with new ways of thinking.

I remember Dr. Simonton's words, which inspired me and gave me hope: "We can use our imagination to influence our thoughts in a healthy direction, thus increasing our health."

We have the ability to restore our health. We can consciously use our imagination to influence our thoughts with healthy images and increase our health. As our awareness grows, we can use a variety of psychological tools to release the blockages that have created disease. As the issues from our past are owned and resolved, the emotions calm down and the immune system strengthens. *The body then knows how to heal itself.*

Page 18 of the *Getting Well Audio Program Guidebook* tells us how this takes place:

> "The cycle of cancer development can be reversed. The pathways by which feelings can be translated into physiological conditions conducive to cancer growth can also be used to restore health...

> "It is particularly important that there be a change either in patients' perceptions of themselves—so they believe they can solve whatever life problems faced them before the onset of the cancer, or in their perceptions of their problems—so they believe they can cope with them more effectively.

> "The results of patients' beliefs in their opportunities for recovery, coupled with their 're-decision' about the problems they face, are an approach to life that includes hope and anticipation. Altered feelings of hope and anticipation are recorded in the limbic system, just as were the previous feelings of hopelessness and despair. Once these feelings are recorded in the limbic system, messages are sent to the hypothalamus reflecting the altered emotional state—a state that includes an increased will to live. The

hypothalamus then sends messages to the pituitary gland that reflect the altered emotional state.

"The hypothalamus in turn reverses the suppression of the immune system, so that the body's defenses once again mobilize against abnormal cells. The pituitary gland (which is part of the endocrine system), receiving messages from the hypothalamus, sends messages to the rest of the endocrine system, restoring the body's hormonal balance. With balance restored, the body will discontinue producing large numbers of abnormal cells, leaving fewer such cells for either treatment or the body's revitalized defenses to cope with.

"Normal functioning of the immune system and reduced production of abnormal cells create the optimal conditions for cancer regression. Remaining abnormal cells can be destroyed either by treatment or by the body's defenses.

"Patients who have participated in their own recovery often have much greater psychological strength than they had before the disease. From the process of facing a life-threatening illness, confronting basic life issues, and learning their power to influence their health, they emerge not just restored to health, but restored with a sense of potency and control over their lives that they may never have felt before the illness."

Dr. Simonton's two books, *Getting Well Again* and *The Healing Journey*, elaborate further on this self-healing process.

Dr. de Kooker, goes on to say in her article:

"We are not victims of our personality or circumstances....We are able to create new health-enhancing patterns which will shift our focus away from disease and toward living fully."

When we change our attitude from toxic to healing, we can create health. Just as our self-sabotaging decisions cause constant stress and eventually disable the immune system, when we change those toxic attitudes to healing decisions, the mind and emotions relax and become peaceful. This activates the parasympathetic nervous system, which enables the pituitary, hypothalamus, and adrenal glands to release chemicals and hormones that strengthen the immune system and heal the body. Therefore, attitude is everything.

The Power of Attitude

Our subconscious attitudes dictate the outcome of our lives and our health. Attitude affects whether surgery, chemotherapy, drugs, diet, or any form of healing will be successful or detrimental to the body. Norman Cousins, author of *Anatomy of an Illness*, added many years to his life by using humor to change his attitude. He said that drugs are not always necessary; however, belief in the treatment is. A physician I know always tells her cancer patients when they ask her if they should have surgery, "If you believe in it, do it. If you don't believe in it, it will not be successful for you."

Let's look at the effect of attitude on diet. Good examples of this can be found in the studies done on centenarians, people who live past the age of 100. One man studied drank a bottle of scotch whiskey a day and claimed that it was responsible for him living longer than 100 years. Another woman attributed her long-lived healthy life to eating a dozen eggs every day along with a half-pound of bacon. Even though both these people broke cardinal rules of modern nutrition, their attitude about what they were consuming was stronger than the effects of the alcohol or cholesterol. When Jesus was asked by his disciples what food they should eat, He told them that it's not what we put into our mouths that poisons us, it's what comes out that causes the problems. Our own words and attitudes can kill us.

My attitude as a cancer patient before I took my mind, thoughts, and feelings into my own hands was that there was something wrong with me. I was holding onto a toxic attitude of "others are right, therefore I must be wrong."

Growing up, I was often blamed for others' mistakes. I dared not correct them because then the attacks became more vicious. I helped others survive by taking on the blame. I remember thinking as a child that if I yelled back the way I was yelled at, they wouldn't survive.

I was frightened by anger, as growing up in the midst of war showed me that anger could kill. I saw members of my family become hysterical, prone to irrational attacks that were subconscious behavior patterns they'd learned to survive. Ever notice the horrible things that come out of people's mouths when they are angry? They say hurtful things that have nothing to do with the truth.

As a child, I thought that I had no choice but to give in because I loved my family deeply and wanted them to survive. I also knew that I would be viciously attacked, verbally and physically, if I dared a confrontation. I now understand that it was not done maliciously, but simply out of not knowing a better way. This is how they were treated and they, in turn, treated others the same way. I resolved not to be that way, but did not know how to make decisions that reflected my best interests.

One of the physical causes of cancer is the body attacking itself by growing abnormal cells. Years later when I was criticized and attacked by a coworker—just as my family had done to me growing up—I blamed myself for not being good enough. That dose of self-blame was a form of attack on my own well-being. I believe that was the onset of my cancer.

Attitudes of Cancer Patients and the Effect on the Body

I have found in my work with cancer clients that they have a pattern of attacking themselves—just as the body attacks itself by growing abnormal cells—by self-blame and making decisions against the self. The attitude of cancer patients is that prior experience has shown them that aggressive people cannot be corrected easily without an all-out war or viciousness that is totally unacceptable. Wanting to maintain peace, they give in and suppress their anger. *Cancer patients want to maintain peace at any price.* They swallow blame in order to maintain the peace, not knowing that blame stored in the body is like poison, not realizing there is a healthier solution.

Swallowing blame and suppressing anger was an important defense mechanism in childhood; giving in was probably necessary for survival. As we grow up, however, it becomes essential to reverse that process and develop self-worth and self-expression skills that allow us to be treated fairly and with respect. Spending time alone is very helpful for regaining your ability to see things accurately, for reclaiming your self, and for making decisions that take care of your self, which energizes your body, mind, and spirit.

In addition, just as I thought I had no worth as a woman, most cancer patients get their sense of self-worth and love by nurturing others instead of valuing and loving themselves. This is a common theme among the thousands of people I have worked with from all walks of life. Even billionaires, millionaires, celebrities, royalty, physicians, professionals of all kinds, businessmen, artists, housewives, you name it, all feel this way. I have seen it over and over with each person I worked with. They all had a similar toxic attitude of feeling "not good enough" that was being held in the body, creating disease.

Another usual attitude of cancer patients I have worked with is: "This cancer will kill me, and there is nothing I can do. It is because of my genetic inheritance...or the poisonous environment...or a punishment. I must have done something terrible to deserve this. God is punishing me. Cancer is death and nothing will help—certainly not changing my attitudes. That has nothing to do with my cancer. It is only a matter of time before I will die a horrible, painful death."

These attitudes are debilitating and make the cancer progress much faster. It is a self-fulfilling prophecy. The more patients allow these thoughts to be their mindset, the more the cancer progresses. There are well-known cases in which a doctor has told a patient, "You have only three to six months to live." That thought is so invasive and produces such a deep belief in the doctor's words that these people usually die within that time period. Family members then say, "You see, the doctor was right."

Some doctors are now learning to phrase what they say so that it gives a measure of hope to the patient. A more accurate way of communicating the diagnosis to the patient is to say, "According to statistics, 95 percent of patients with a similar condition die within three to six months. Some recover and have a spontaneous remission. You may be one of these people in the 5-percent bracket who survive and get well."

There are well-known research studies that demonstrate the power of belief using the placebo effect. One study described in detail in Dr. Simonton's audiotape program, *Getting Well*, was done by Dr. Bruno Klopfer, who invited a terminal patient to try a new experimental drug called krobiacin. This patient's hope was rekindled and with much enthusiasm, he told Dr. Klopfer that he knew this drug would save his life. All the patients who received this drug showed that it had no effect on their cancer—*except this patient who knew it would save his life.* He recovered from cancer.

An article later came out in the newspaper confirming that krobiacin was found to be useless in curing cancer. When this patient saw this article, he became so disheartened that his cancer reappeared. Dr. Klopfer noticed what happened and decided to bring this patient back for another experiment. He told the physicians to talk enthusiastically about the "new" krobiacin that just arrived and then invited the patient to witness this event. "It is a lot stronger and has a better shelf-life," they explained with much excitement. The hopes of this patient were once more rekindled. Dr. Klopfer gave the patient a sugar pill. The patient recovered from his cancer a lot faster this time.

Unfortunately, another article in the newspaper confirmed once more that krobiacin had been discarded as a total failure in the treatment of cancer. After the patient saw that article, his cancer returned and he died.

Changing Toxic Attitudes to Healing Attitudes

When we change our attitude, we change our state of health. Just as our harmful beliefs and attitudes can create disease, we can create health by changing our attitude. As we reverse our toxic attitudes, we reverse our cancer.

Deepak Chopra, the well-known author of *Quantum Healing,* tells of his own experience of seeing belief heal. When he was a doctor at Massachusetts General Hospital, the daughter of a terminal cancer patient in that hospital asked him if he would give her mother a clean bill of health. Because he knew the patient was dying anyway, he believed there would be no harm in tellng this woman that she was fine. He did so and thought no more about it.

A year later this same woman, whom he thought would have died from cancer soon after he last saw her, showed up in the hospital looking very healthy. After recovering from shock, he asked her why she was there. She said, "Well, doctor, I thought I should come back for a checkup." When he asked her how she was, she said, "In the beginning, I had a lot of pain, but I just kept remembering what you said—that I was fine. So I would remind myself each day that I was fine. I decided that the pain must be in my mind. After a while, it went away."

Dr. Chopra told her, "Whatever you are doing is obviously working, so just continue it." It was the beginning of Dr. Chopra's understanding that there was more to healing than just drugs and surgery.

Attitude alone can heal. When this patient changed her attitude from "dying of cancer" to "being fine," she healed. I have learned this from my own experience as well as with my students. *We have the ability to persuade the mind to adopt healthy healing perceptions that produce wellness images in the brain and rebuild the immune system, creating health.*

For example, when I began my self-healing program, I worked daily practicing changing my toxic attitudes to new healthy attitudes. After deep relaxation, I visualized myself already believing these new attitudes and living my life accordingly. I would envision myself in situations in my life from the new, healthy, empowered perspective rather than from the old, toxic disempowered perspective. Incidents that made me upset in the past, I was now able to see in a new light, feeling calm, peaceful, and quiet inside, feeling good about myself and my life.

As I practiced these new healing attitudes sincerely for several days, I noticed how my pain diminished. The more I was able to experience these new attitudes as real, valid, true, desirable, and solid within me, the more joy I felt inside. The effect on my body was quite amazing. As I observed the changes in my physical sensations—pain disappearing, strange physical symptoms dissolving, and good feelings returning—my energy grew, and my functioning rapidly improved.

That was when I knew *it is the attitudes and the emotions they produce that heal, not the food I eat or the vitamins I take.* I celebrated with a cup of coffee. I was so convinced of the power of attitude that I allowed myself to indulge in whatever gave me joy. I understood that the feelings of pleasure were far more important than the caffeine I was putting into my body. I knew pleasure and joy were being registered in my brain, which was releasing healing chemicals and hormones that were strengthening my immune system. It was the beginning of reversing my cancer and returning to health.

I find attitude to be the cornerstone of most, if not all, problems in life—physical, emotional, mental, and spiritual. The views that we hold about ourselves, our bodies, our health, our life, other people, a higher power, and the world affect our lives dramatically.

Our attitude either heals us or makes us sick. When a person is hopeful and enthusiastic about his or her form of treatment, it can heal. However, the treatment is not what heals, it is the patient's hopeful, enthusiastic attitude that releases health-building chemicals that allows the body to heal itself.

In Part II you will discover your own self-sabotaging attitudes that caused your disease and learn how to create healing attitudes, which will release healing chemicals in the body that strengthen the immune system and restore health.

In this chapter, we have looked at the psychological causes of disease. In the next chapter, you will learn from my own journey with cancer the importance of taking care of your psychological needs that, if ignored, will lead to disease.

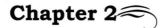
Learning From My Journey With Cancer

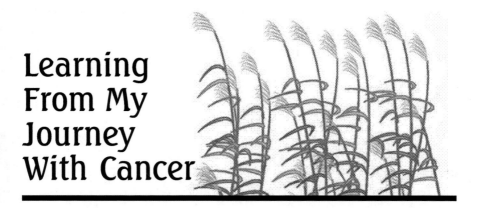

I know the terror of cancer first hand. I have been diagnosed with cancer three times. By the third time, I just couldn't face another round of surgery and chemotherapy, which had left me so debilitated that I couldn't make a simple phone call. I feared that if I went to the hospital again, I was going to die. I decided to give myself three months to practice what I had been teaching others for many years, combining ageless wisdom with the latest scientific research in mind/body medicine.

I synthesized all that I had learned from psychoneuroimmunology and psychology from Western culture and healing imagery and techniques from the East into a simple method. Within three months my tumor shrank to half its former size. Eight months later, I returned to radiant health. At the completion of my self-healing program, the doctor examined me. "A miracle has happened, your cancer is gone!" he said in amazement.

"It's not a miracle, doctor," I replied. "I have been practicing self-healing for an hour three times a day. If I can do it, anyone can." That was in 1995, and I remain in radiant health to this day.

In August 1992, I was first diagnosed with aggressive breast cancer. It was a total shock to find out that cancer was lurking in my body without my knowledge. I started losing hope, felt discouraged, and began doubting everything I had learned and had been teaching for so many years. Maybe my healing work was just a placebo or some kind of hypnosis that I didn't understand. From time to time, a part of me would observe the drama with disbelief. Should I have my breast removed, or should I trust that I can heal the cancer myself? I was confused.

A close friend of mine died of breast cancer because she neglected to have the tumor removed in time, and it spread to her lymph nodes. That memory kept nagging me to follow the traditional medical route.

My good friend from Colorado warned me, "Don't follow the popular medical treatment. You are a healer; you can heal yourself. Don't buy into the illusion of cancer."

I wanted so much to believe her. She recommended that I see an American Indian Shaman in Alberta. I took the next flight to Canada.

Looking for Alternative Answers

The Shaman told me that he first planned to take me to a sweat lodge and that if it did not work, then it would be necessary to visit a private sweat lodge in a more high-energy location. Being around him was an adventure; he was so wise and seemed to be able to read my thoughts clearly. I started feeling hopeful and good about myself for plunging in and taking on this new experience.

A woman with breast cancer of several years was waiting in line with me for the sweat lodge. "Has it helped you?" I asked her. "Is your cancer gone?" "It's better, but I still have it," she replied. "Has it helped other women?" "Yes, it helped some women." "How long does it take?" I asked. "We don't know for sure," she responded.

The Shaman approached me saying, "If you see blue light, then that means that you will heal; if you see red light, that means that there is nothing that can be done to help you." I started shaking inside. *What if I see red light?* My anxiety started rising. I had to wait for several hours before the sweat lodge was ready. It felt like I was waiting for judgment day, whether I was to live or die. "You don't have to believe it if you don't want to," I said to myself.

When I spoke with my friend, she told me, "You must have faith or else it doesn't work." "But I don't have faith; how do I make myself have faith?" I asked her. "Pray to have faith," she responded. I prayed to have faith and tried hard to do that. "I can create it to be blue. Even if it's red, I will change it to blue," I resolved.

Inside the sweat lodge, it was dark and steaming hot. I was watching intently to see what color showed up. For an instant, I thought I saw red. I quickly turned it to blue, but I wasn't sure. I started shaking again. "Did you see red or blue?" I asked the Shaman. He looked at me and asked me what I saw. "Blue," I responded. He stared at me without saying a word. I started shaking again.

"I'm not going to let myself get affected by this...maybe its all nonsense," I said, trying to reassure myself. "We have to do another sweat lodge in a private place," the Shaman informed me. My panic intensified. "It's a sacrifice on the Shaman's part," explained my friend. "He has to sacrifice a part of his life in order to heal you." "I don't want him to sacrifice anything for me," I declared. I packed my bags and left.

Now believing that surgery was the only solution, I thought to myself, "It's only a breast. Maybe it's a lesson in detachment." I decided to have the mastectomy.

The hospital was a nightmare, so cold and impersonal. It looked like I had entered a torture chamber in a concentration camp. The butchers were ready to cut me up. A woman waiting for her surgery had tears of despair in her eyes. My eyes met hers and started burning with terror—that deep pain of awaiting a possible death sentence. At one point, I thought I saw a dark angel of death facing me. I sent him love, and the image disappeared.

The anesthetic dosage felt too much for my light body. I could barely recover my breath. "Breathe, Goodman, breathe," I kept hearing the doctor command sternly. I found it so difficult to keep on breathing. It was such hard work, almost impossible to do. Horrible torturous nausea overcame me every time I tried to move my eyes even slightly. Am I dying now? A very faint part of me was witnessing and observing silently. When I finally opened my eyes, my husband and son were staring at me in the recovery room. "I am alive," I thought. I tried to smile. Nausea overwhelmed me. "Don't move," I told myself.

"Two out of 19 lymph nodes removed were affected," the doctor informed me. "Chemotherapy starts next week, and you will need it for a year." The prognosis was a 50-percent chance of recovery with chemotherapy.

"Don't do chemotherapy," warned my friend "That can kill you. And it is much more difficult to heal naturally if you do it. Instead, go to Boston and try Ann Wigmore's wheat grass juicing. Many people have healed themselves using that method."

"Yes, you could wait three weeks to start treatment," my oncologist said.

"Anything but chemotherapy," I thought—and took the train to Boston.

The wheat grass juice made me nauseous, and I kept throwing up, but the stories of success kept me going and gave me hope. The instructor said, "A live-food diet is the answer." Yet I found it so difficult to digest. It was tasteless and repulsive to me. I knew I must learn to love it if I wanted to stay alive.

"You must stay on this diet for the rest of your life, or you will die," is what I heard from many of the participants—who looked green to me. I watched a video of a physician who healed his cancer using this diet. But two months after he stopped and started eating other foods, he died. My fear emerged again. I kept hearing my thoughts buzzing inside my head: "I literally can't stomach this diet...it makes me sick. But if I don't do it, I will die."

I saw people eating delicious food in restaurants. It smelled and looked so good. I felt deep depression envelop me—I could never enjoy these foods again. "How is it possible that so many people are eating this poisonous food, yet they look so healthy?" I kept wondering. I saw someone eating lentil soup; I craved it so much that I buckled under and had a cup. It never tasted more delicious. I felt happy, satisfied, and reluctantly left the clinic against the advice of the teachers who felt I was committing suicide.

I began chemo, the recommended formula called 5FU. I reacted to it very strongly. Besides throwing up all the time, my thoughts became clouded, and I was sure the drugs were affecting my brain. Most of my hair fell out, and after eight treatments, severe symptoms of menopause began.

Two of my older sisters came from Israel to help me manage during chemotherapy. My sisters were wonderful. One stroked my face while the chemotherapy was flowing into my veins. Tears were rolling down my cheeks, yet it was so good to feel her love. She had never stroked my face before. "So having cancer is what it takes to feel my sister's love," I thought, remembering our conflicted childhood. Feeling nauseous in the car, I started panicking, and my sister comforted me.

At home, the effects of the chemo intensified. My body felt invaded by a horrible combat, one that was killing me from within, stripping away my defenses. It felt like I was being bombarded with machine guns inside my body, like total destruction was taking place. The agony was unbearable. My brain was badly affected. I could barely function, and I became paranoid and started thinking bizarre thoughts and speaking strangely. It frightened my husband and sisters, and it frightened me as well. The throwing up seemed neverending. "This is the worst of tortures," I thought, "but I must obey and be tortured or else I will die."

Every time I thought of chemotherapy, I felt nauseous. "I don't want to do chemo, but I must," I cried, while speaking to the participants at a workshop I was attending. "You don't have to if you don't want to," someone told me.

"But you don't understand—I have no choice. I will die if I don't follow the traditional medical route."

"It's your choice," I vaguely remember someone saying. "I *wish* it were my choice; I have no choice. I don't have the courage to refuse it." I knew this was true, even though I was feeling sick at the idea of forcing myself to enter the torture chamber again.

Forging a New Path

A well-known doctor was giving a workshop on cancer in Boston. I begged my son and my husband, who was a total skeptic of therapy and self-healing, to go with me. They finally agreed.

It was a disaster. We left overcome with depression. Instead of feeling encouraged, we felt doomed. On top of my despair, I felt guilty for dragging them along. All that money, time, and energy just to come away feeling that there was no hope.

Next, I went to the Macrobiotic Center to study the macrobiotic philosophy of eating and to give this diet a try. At the center, I heard stories of people who had healed from cancer. "But those who stopped the diet, their tumors came back bigger with a vengeance," one teacher said. I was once more longing to eat regular food, but again was too frightened to stop the diet. I was able to maintain this diet for a longer period of time than the live-food diet, but I eventually did give it up.

I underwent chemotherapy every three weeks, exploring as many alternative therapies as I could in between treatments. One therapist, who specialized in systematic desensitization for chemotherapy, was helpful in reducing some of the side effects, especially the nausea I felt every time the thought of chemotherapy or an image of the hospital or the doctor passed through my mind. One friend didn't want to accompany me to the chemo treatment. "I don't want you to associate me with chemotherapy," she said. I was able to keep my private practice as a psychologist going by cutting my hours to a minimum.

Before the eighth treatment of chemotherapy, in December 1992, I cried hysterically, refusing to go for treatment. I cried the whole day, but finally forced myself to go against my will. "You really don't want to do it," said a close friend who accompanied me to my treatment. "No," I agreed, my eyes burning with tears, "but I have no choice."

After that chemo treatment, my period stopped abruptly, and I started having hot flashes and many strange symptoms that scared me immensely. I became dysfunctional and found any small task to be a huge undertaking. Even a simple conversation or making a phone call was traumatic. Often I would think, "Cancer has taken over and spread; that's why I'm feeling so strange." Fear would intensify the symptoms, and the disease became worse.

A woman who'd healed herself of cancer told me about a program in Los Angeles. "I'm not wasting any more time and money," I told her. "You must do this program if you don't want a reoccurrence," she persisted.

"Three thousand dollars!" my husband shouted, "That's a waste of money. It's not going to help." "It's my life and I am worth more than $3,000. I'm going," I said. "I'd like you to come with me to be my support person."

His boss convinced him that he should go.

Something to Believe In

In Dr. Carl Simonton's seminar in Los Angeles, I sighed with relief as I heard the following words:

> "Research has shown the common ingredient of why some people heal from cancer and others don't to be 'belief.' Why do some people heal from chemotherapy and others don't? Why does a macrobiotic diet or whatever help some, while others die? People who believe that something will help them feel 'hope' and the enthusiasm that accompanies that feeling. This enthusiasm registers in the brain, and the brain then releases chemicals and hormones that strengthen the immune system. The body then knows how to heal itself. What we need to do is quiet ourselves and get out of the way. We don't even need to know what's wrong."

I jumped with joy; I had found the answer. All I have to do is strengthen my belief in my ability to find the way to heal myself. I can choose to believe whatever I want. As long as I believe it, it will work. I can practice believing whatever I wish, and within two to three months, I will change accordingly.

"It takes about six to eight weeks to change an old belief to a new belief, with regular motivated practice," we were told. These words were like precious gems to me. After two days of spending time with this program, most of my symptoms disappeared, and I started smiling again. I not only had hope, but my faith was restored.

At one point during the seminar, I was crying hysterically, asking my husband to help me gather the courage to stop chemotherapy. I was so weak and wounded from those treatments. I begged the teachers to give me permission to stop treatments. They refused to take that kind of responsibility saying, "That's a good question to take to your inner wisdom and hear the answer from within."

I tried asking my wisdom, but all I got back was a terrible fear at the thought of having to continue this torture as soon as I returned home.

After crying intensely, I was approached by one teacher who said, "It is obvious." "What is obvious?" I asked, puzzled. "Your body is giving you the answer very powerfully. Look how you are crying." "What answer? You mean my crying is telling me that it is okay to stop chemotherapy?" I wanted someone to say to me, "Yes, it's okay to stop." No one dared say these words to me except this courageous teacher. "It is obvious what your body is saying to you. These are the signs from your inner wisdom. They come with a strong feeling."

I was still not sure what the message was. However, when I returned home, I stopped chemotherapy. I believe that if I had continued treatments, I would have become totally dysfunctional. I am so happy that I had the courage to stop even though it terrified me to do so.

In July 1993, I received another shocking blow. A cancerous tumor appeared in my right breast. The new tumor was about one centimeter this time and a different form of cancer, not as aggressive as the previous attack. I was devastated because I thought I was getting better. Feelings of despair started creeping in and strange symptoms reappeared. I refused the recommended mastectomy and angrily left my surgeon to work with another surgeon who agreed that lumpectomy would be sufficient. I refused chemotherapy, radiation, and medication.

"I don't understand why chemotherapy did not get rid of this tumor," my new female surgeon exclaimed. My new male oncologist told me initially that six months of chemotherapy was sufficient. When I told my oncologist that I decided to stop chemotherapy after the eighth session, he revealed to me that some research had shown that eight sessions of 5FU were sufficient. That was helpful to know. However, if I had known that earlier, it would have spared me a lot of pain.

I studied with a healing master who taught me that it is important to monitor chemotherapy to the level of T cell production in the body and not to just give the same dosage to everyone. I remembered telling my first oncologist that the dosage was too high for me, that my body was too light to handle that amount of chemicals. I'd hardly ever taken any medications before. I explained to him how my brain could barely function. My oncologist's response was that it was the right amount for my body weight. "It is only emotional anxiety," he had insisted.

Luckily, I was able to stop treatments. Later on, I heard that a friend who was on chemotherapy became a vegetable—she lost her functioning ability completely. My inner knowing stopped me from becoming a vegetable just in time. I wish I had paid attention to the signals my body was giving me and stopped earlier.

There were times when my fear started getting out of control. I had terrible panic attacks at night. My body would jump in bed in terror. I used to be an expert in treating people with panic attacks and had developed numerous techniques that helped many people. None of these techniques helped me until I looked inside and identified the beliefs that were causing my terror.

"What are your beliefs?" I asked myself. "I don't know. It is just terrifying to die, I guess." I heard a faint response. I guided myself to feel the terror and exaggerate it, as I had often guided my clients in Gestalt therapy. I started crying, connecting with that energy of fear. I allowed myself to regress to the feelings of a little girl. As I was crying, several beliefs came out of my mouth in a row. One of those beliefs was, "I am dying all alone, and no one can come with me. I don't know where I am going, and it's terrifying to leave everything and go alone into nowhere."

"Aha, so that's what you believe," I responded to myself, suddenly feeling calm. I realized that as soon as I identified the underlying beliefs that caused the terror, the terror disappeared. I then changed them to new healing decisions, such as "I can choose to die in perfect health at an age when I am sure that I have finished my work on earth, and with a feeling of fulfillment and satisfaction." My panic attacks disappeared, and I started sleeping well at night.

Making Major Changes

"Cancer is a signpost so that we can make changes," said Dr. Lawrence Le Shan, author of *Cancer as a Turning Point*. I kept contemplating that statement. I started making changes in my life. I stopped working full time and cut down my hours to just a few a week. I stayed with my friends in Colorado for a few weeks at a time and visited my family in Israel.

I began noticing that when I was in Colorado, I was feeling much better. But as soon as I returned home, my body started deteriorating so fast, it seemed like it was decaying in front of my eyes. "What is it? What is happening?" I kept on asking myself. "Maybe the cancer is progressing, and I am dying," I would often think with a pang of fear. Every little pain or symptom was a terrifying sign that cancer had returned.

"Cancer is death." Everyone knew that, and sometimes so did I. It was so difficult to change that belief.

When I was in Israel, I noticed that I started to feel better again, and cancer became a joke. Of course I can beat it! Then I would come back home to New Jersey and, immediately, strange symptoms would develop. I would feel fear and hopelessness, as though my home was stimulating a response in me of cancer and death.

On the next journey to Israel, once more I started feeling better. I gathered enough courage and told my husband that I was not returning home to New Jersey. I decided to spend six months in Colorado and six months in Israel. I told my husband that if he wished to join me, he was welcome, and if not, whatever he wanted to do I would always love him and be his good friend. He responded by saying, "You are not giving me much choice. I don't want to leave New Jersey. What good is our marriage if I am here and you are there?"

"What good is our marriage if I am there and I am dead?" I said. "If you want to get a divorce, that's up to you." I continued, "In three years, you are planning to retire anyway, so if you want to join me in three years, you are welcome." "I'll think about it," he responded.

Two days later my husband called and said that he'd decided to get a divorce. I was shaking with fear for half an hour, thinking, "What if my cancer gets worse, and I'm in a wheelchair? Who will take care of me after 32 years of marriage?"

"That's no reason to stay married," a quiet voice within me responded. "I'd rather die, kill myself, than have him suffer wheeling me around and becoming enslaved to my sickness."

Feeling resolved that this was the right thing to do I suddenly experienced a surge of excitement. "I'm free! Oh my God, I'm free to do as I please without having to compromise or feel guilty about living life according to my heart's desires. I should have done it 31 years ago." Life had turned into an exciting adventure.

However, the chemotherapy damage was not completely healed. Every little stress overwhelmed my fragile nervous system. It has taken me years to recover from the effects of the chemotherapy and regain my full strength and stamina.

In August 1994, I returned to New Jersey for our divorce and to move my belongings to Colorado. "Give me one year to leave some of my stuff here," I asked my ex-husband. He agreed. Once more being back in New Jersey in those familiar surroundings, my strange symptoms reappeared. Having to throw many things away and finding it extremely difficult to decide what to move from my huge home—filled with books, tapes, videos, and treasured objects—to Colorado added enormous stress to my already overtaxed body.

Four months later, in December 1994, my doctor confirmed my fear that cancer had returned—the worst attack ever. We both "knew" that cancer had spread everywhere, and I was dying. "You must go to the hospital right away," he said with a grim expression. I had a 4- to 5-centimeter hard tumor in my breast, swollen lymph nodes, plus strange symptoms that scared me, and pain in many parts of my body, especially my bones.

"I tried everything and nothing worked," I said to myself. "I have no choice but to go the medical route." I'd completely overlooked how in the past I'd gotten better and worse, better and worse—according to what was happening in my life. I lost hope and gave up. I made arrangements to go to the hospital in Colorado right away.

Suddenly I burst out crying hysterically. I started a dialogue with my inner self as I had been teaching my clients to do for the past 20 years as a Gestalt therapist. "Why are you crying so hysterically?" I asked.

I heard a disembodied voice within me respond, "I'm so afraid for you. If you go to the hospital, you will die in a few weeks. They will cut another piece and another piece, and then poison me with chemotherapy, radiation, and all kinds of medications, not meaning to kill you, but that is what will happen. You will be too frightened and weak and forget that you can heal yourself. You won't have the strength to connect and listen to me— your inner voice. Others' thought patterns and opinions will be easily imprinted in your mind, and it will take too much effort to trust your own knowing."

"But I have no choice," I responded intently. "I have tried everything and it did not work. The hospital is the only solution now. The cancer will kill me if I don't get it cut out."

"Do you want to go to the hospital?" I heard a firm part of me inquire.

"No, of course I don't want to go to the hospital," I said indignantly.

"Then you don't have to do what you don't want to do."

"What do you mean I don't have to? I have no choice," I pleaded.

"Do you want to?" that firm voice continued.

"No....Oh my God, I don't have to go to the hospital if I don't want to! I am free to do as I wish. It is my life, my body. What a relief!"

Heeding My Inner Voice

Immediately my energy perked up as I started repeating with joy, "It's my choice, I can choose. I don't have to listen to what others are dictating that I must do. I don't have to listen to anyone."

"But what should I do now?" I asked myself cautiously.

I thought for a time, then answered, "Give yourself three months to practice everything you have learned and have been teaching. If you don't succeed, you can always go to the hospital then."

"That's a good idea. This way I can put all I have been teaching to the test, to see whether it works or not. Besides, if it's my time to die, I'd much rather die in peace in a fairly healthy body rather than become a zombie who needs others to take care of me."

"Be careful; don't tell anyone about your plan. You know their fear and well-meaning intentions will weaken you, and you may forget this feeling of hope and joy."

I remembered how, when I refused the recommended medical intervention after my lumpectomy, family and friends from all over the world called me to tell me I must have the chemotherapy and radiation and listen to the doctors. People who'd never called me before in the 53 years of my life suddenly felt it was their right or duty to tell me how to live my life. Their fear weakened me immensely, just as the people who were positive and nurturing strengthened me.

This time I told no one. I was so weak from the illness and all the fears that came with it; I knew that they would be able to influence me, and I would give in and end up going to the hospital, which I knew would be my death.

I started feeling shaky as I picked up the phone to cancel my hospitalization. "You are risking your life, probably committing suicide," said the doctor on the other end of the phone.

I started shaking. Fear surged up again. "How dare I tell the doctor that I can do what I feel is best for me, that I have a right to decide how I wish to live my life? How dare I doubt what he recommends that I do?" I almost caved in. I remembered how afraid I was of doctors most of my life growing up, thinking they were gods and that I must never oppose what they say.

I gathered courage and said, "I will think about it," and quickly hung up the phone. My heart started pounding with fear.

"You don't have to give so much power to doctors if you don't want to," I heard a faint voice console me. I decided not to tell anyone what I was doing and booked a flight to Hawaii to be alone.

"Should I at least have a biopsy?" I asked myself.

I heard a definite "No! What for? The needle will make the tumor bleed and the cancer will spread faster. It will be much more difficult to heal it then."

I also knew that what the doctors tell me gets imprinted deep into my consciousness and subconscious mind. Changing those imprints would take up too much of my energy. That energy is too precious and needs to be devoted to the healing imagery.

The next day I woke up in disbelief thinking, "Me? Cancer? No way! I am not buying into that illusion." I leaped out of bed and went outside to jump on my trampoline. I was so weak and had so much pain that I could hardly climb up on it. I jumped gently, affirming over and over with each jump, *"I am getting stronger and stronger, healthier and healthier, happier and happier, wiser and wiser every day."*

That sentence has been very helpful to me. I learned it when I was in despair and feeling hopeless, knowing that death was imminent and that it could show up at any moment. It rekindled a spark of hope in me, which eventually helped me get back on my feet.

On the way to Hawaii, I had stopped in Los Angeles and San Francisco to attend several workshops, where I learned ancient Chinese Healing Tao exercises. I was driving from Los Angeles to San Francisco feeling very anxious about so many hours behind the wheel, wondering whether my body could handle it. I started practicing some of the exercises I'd just learned in the workshop in Los Angeles. I visualized my internal organs smiling. To my surprise, they energized me, and the journey ended up being quite easy. "I'm on the right track," I congratulated myself.

In Hawaii, being alone was very difficult at first. "Face your loneliness, feel the pain, don't run away from it," I remember telling myself. For a few days, I stayed in bed crying, delving deep into my pain. I was terrified of becoming dysfunctional from so much pain. My fear was of dying an awful torturous death with intolerable pain. I couldn't bare the thought that some person might have to take care of me. I was very tempted to call someone, to connect and talk with my family and friends. I refrained and forced myself to face my pain full-blown. I was so scared that the pain would get worse, that it would be too much for me to bear. After several days of wallowing and feeling my pain, it suddenly vanished.

I practiced self-healing three times a day—doing deep relaxation, changing my unhealthy attitudes to new healing perceptions, seeing my internal organs smiling, and integrating all that I had learned. I devoted about three hours a day to this work—an hour in the morning, another hour at noon, and an hour in the evening.

I started feeling so good, with a lot of renewed energy, that a definite spark of hope emerged. "There is no way I am dying if I feel this good," I said with joy, smiling at myself in the mirror. "Well done, you are on the right track." I celebrated with a cup of coffee. After having tried so many strict diets of organic food, macrobiotic food, live food, wheat grass, and vegetable juicing, I became aware that health and healing is not so much about what I eat, but more about what self-sabotaging attitudes "eat" me.

The journey was not smooth. There were times I would forget, overload myself with work, get overstressed, and any new symptom, a faint new pain, would bring back full-blown strange symptoms that said, "Cancer is back."

I didn't realize that the strange symptoms I experienced in my body were because of these attitudes. I became fearful that cancer had spread. The fear, "I have tried everything and nothing has helped; cancer is spreading, and soon I will die an unspeakable, painful death" was a common thought process that often passed through me. I had no idea that it was the attitudes that created the pain. These painful symptoms and the emotional discomfort I was feeling were the body's way of showing me my unhealthy attitudes.

I noticed how sensitive my body became to other people's energies and their negative thoughts. I started paying more attention to the people I associated with and the places I went. Even a visit to the supermarket could drain my energy, and I would come back home feeling exhausted. I had to learn to cut down on a lot of my activities and take more time to be alone and in nature. I learned to pay attention and follow the body's feedback system, which took time, diligence, and focus.

Three months later, I returned to Israel. I went to a local doctor to find out how my cancer was doing. "I have not followed the medical route," I told him, "but I would like to have an objective opinion. I feel that my tumor has shrunk. But I don't know if I am biased, so a neutral diagnosis by you would be appreciated."

"Why should I examine you if you won't follow my recommendation?" he asked.

I thought for a moment. "If you think that it is still dangerous, then I promise that I'll drop everything from my life and practice the self-healing techniques full time."

Remember these words, I said to myself. *You will drop everything and continue practicing your self-healing full time!*

I was amazed at how easily I'd lost my discipline of practicing what was so helpful to me.

"Okay," he said and agreed to examine me.

"Yes, it is dangerous," the doctor told me after the examination. "You must go to the hospital right away."

"How large is the tumor?" I asked with a sinking heart.

"About 2 to 2 1/2 centimeters. It is very hard and yes, it is cancer," he said.

I sighed with relief. "I'm on the right track. It shrank down to half its size," I explained with delight. "How are the lymph nodes? Are they still swollen?" I continued, feeling apprehensive.

"The lymph nodes are normal," he said.

I couldn't contain my smile of relief, "Thank you, bless you."

"Remember to drop everything," I reminded myself. I wondered if I could do that. Would I do it? It was so difficult. I was sure I'd keep thinking, "I can't drop this" and "I have to do that" and on and on. I now believe that if I'd had the courage to drop everything, I would have healed a lot faster.

I did continue practicing my self-healing, although many thoughts came my way that distracted my focus and attention. The doctor's certainty of my cancer and that it was endangering my life shook me very badly. I became more aware of how the thoughts I was holding onto affected me. Once more, I started feeling the strange symptoms. Every little stress was magnified into a huge trauma. My health was deteriorating. "Don't listen to the doctors," I told myself as I tried desperately to erase his diagnosis from my mind. I redoubled my efforts to focus on thoughts that were healing.

Eight months later, in November 1995, my doctor in Colorado told me that my cancer was gone. My surgeon in New York City confirmed, "Your breast is normal."

As recommended, I visited many doctors for checkups every six months in Israel and the United States. Once, when the doctor was running late, I started feeling impatient. As I gazed around the waiting room filled with sick patients, I asked myself, "Since my attitudes create my health, what am I doing sitting here? Why am I spending my time in this way? Isn't there something else I would rather do with this time?" I reflected. "What would I rather choose to do with my time instead of waiting in doctors' offices?

"I would prefer to swim with dolphins, to help people heal themselves, to visit my family in Israel more often, spend time with friends, and do fun things that give me joy," I responded.

"Then do it!" I heard myself say with resolve.

"*But I have to get my blood tested and—*"

"Do you really want to waste time here waiting impatiently for doctors' verdicts?"

I stopped arguing, recalling what I knew deep inside. "No, I would rather do other things. I don't have to force myself to do anything I don't want to do. I know I can heal myself. I don't need the doctor's approval or disapproval." I got up and left the office.

I haven't been to a doctor's office in a long time. Now I listen and respond to my body's signals constantly. *And* I make creating health the highest priority in my life.

Here in this chapter, I have shared my journey to help you in your own recovery or prevention. In the next chapter, we will explore the spiritual causes of cancer and how denial of our inherent goodness and worthiness causes the body to break down. We will also talk about the feedback our symptoms give us that, if understood, can guide us in our healing.

Chapter 3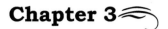

Seeing Your Symptoms as Feedback

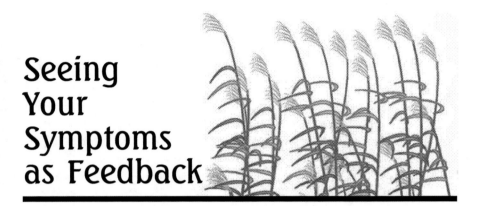

Even though I'd been able to help many people heal from cancer long before my own cancer showed up, when *I* began receiving the early warning signs, I wasn't paying attention. I continued to make decisions that were not in my best interest, which further damaged my health.

In 1991, my husband and I went to Hawaii for a week's vacation. The night before our return home, we were gazing at the beautiful sky, and suddenly deep, dark depression engulfed me. "What is this?" I thought. "Aren't I happy to go back home?" I knew the answer was "no."

I turned to my husband. "I think I need a year alone. Being with you triggers my fear of my father. I need to heal this fear, and the best way to do it is to spend time alone."

My husband replied, "If you want to take a year off, then we will get a divorce. And what about your practice? You've built it up so well. Can you risk losing all your clients?"

"I guess you are right," I agreed, then added to myself, *But if I ever get sick, that will be my sign that I must take a sabbatical.*

I had been working so hard my whole life, especially for the past 30 years almost nonstop. My body craved a time-out, but my overly rational mind blocked that information. It didn't occur to me to take a month or even a week off to rest. Instead, I just shut the whole conversation out of my mind.

I thought I had everything anyone could wish for. I was a very successful psychologist who helped hundreds of people on a weekly basis. I was enjoying prestige, prosperity, and close relationships with family and friends. What I did not realize was that *something of deep meaning was missing in my life.*

I know now that it was the spiritual love within—which I had discovered while studying with a master teacher—that had gradually disappeared from my consciousness and my life. This pure love that made me feel radiant, beautiful, peaceful, and blissfully happy had vanished. I was so preoccupied with handling numerous daily tasks, getting caught up with worries of my own and others' difficulties that I had forgotten to follow my inner guide and to trust that knowing.

One year later, I was diagnosed with aggressive breast cancer. Unfortunately, it wasn't until I received my third cancer diagnosis that I finally learned to listen to the feedback I was being given.

Symptoms are messages from the body telling you that what you are thinking, feeling, and doing is making you sick. You are being alerted to the detrimental effect your attitudes and actions are having on the body. It is the body's way of telling you that it is time to make some changes, that it is having difficulty maintaining a strong immune system, and that it needs your assistance. These signals can help you discover and heal the self-sabotaging decisions you've made against yourself.

When we pay attention to this feedback, listen to the wisdom of the body and begin to make decisions that honor ourselves, we can help the body regain harmony and health. When these signals are ignored or numbed with medication, the result is disease. As we continue to ignore the body's natural feedback mechanism, our health further deteriorates.

In my experience, when we are in the grip of disease, our mind/body/spirit system gives us three different kinds of feedback:

What You Are Doing Is Killing Me

First, symptoms tell us that our unhealthy attitudes are having a destructive effect on the body. These symptoms are messages that can help us discover and heal our toxic decisions about the body. If we ignore these signals, the symptoms get worse. It is the body's way of saying, "Stop! What you are doing is killing me!"

Cancer, with its persistent and relentless messages, was the catalyst that finally forced me to change. I hadn't taken a vacation by myself in 30 years. I was stressed and overworked, working seven days a week, as well as being a wife and mother. I was always there for everyone else but rarely for myself. *I needed to be there for myself as well, so that I could take time out for me.*

One of the toxic attitudes underlying breast cancer is "mothering the world" instead of taking care of one's self. We need to take care of our work and our family, but we also need to take care of our self. It took awhile for me to learn to pay attention to what my body was telling me and to start making changes.

When we do pay attention to the signals our body is giving us and give the body what it needs, we become full partners in our recovery. In Part II you will be shown how to work with the body, rather than against it. When I began listening to the wisdom within me and following that wisdom, things began to change.

Listen to the Wisdom Within

Second, symptoms are messages that we are not listening to the wisdom within. Dr. Albert Schweitzer, the noted physician and humanitarian said, "*Within each of us there is a doctor that knows exactly what we need to do in order to get well.*"

We have the wisdom within us to heal ourselves of physical, emotional, and mental challenges. The wisdom of the ages is within the cells of our bodies. It has been passed on to us for generations through our cells. All the wisdom that was our ancestors' is now contained in every fiber of our body. *The body knows what it needs to regain health.* There is a vast intuitive intelligence contained in our mind/body/spirit system, and by tapping it we can be guided in our recovery.

Symptoms remind us to get quiet and listen to that intuitive knowing that will help restore our health. The biggest challenge in the self-healing process is learning not to be affected by others' thoughts and beliefs, but rather taking your guidance from your own inner wisdom. We all have a wise self inside us that knows what is best for our body. In Part II you will be shown how to access this reservoir of wisdom and use it for your own healing.

Denying Your True Self

Third, symptoms are feedback telling us that we are denying our true self, which is pure love, goodness, and joy. Cancer, on some deep level, is a message that we have moved away from the part of us that is good, loving, and lovable. My experience has shown me that disease is a denial at a subconscious level of our inherent goodness, worthiness, and love and an identification of ourselves as being not good or worthy or loving enough. This denial results in feelings of fear and self-doubt that eventually disable the immune system, creating the environment for cancer and other diseases.

Disease is a message that we are not loving ourselves and are denying our goodness, our needs, and our worth. Specifically, when we make decisions based on the attitude that we are not good, loving people, we get out of alignment with our wholeness and the body begins to turn against itself—just as we have. When we make decisions against ourselves, the body then acts on that decision and begins attacking itself—and the process known as cancer or disease begins.

I have come to understand that the body reflects what we believe and feel inside. Depending on how far away we are from our true self, the thought patterns become clustered and block the flow of vital life-force energy. The farther away, the bigger the blockage. They are like knots snarled together. Each unhealthy thought we hold onto becomes another knot, until sickness strikes us in the area of weakness according to the thoughts we have held in the body.

Our self-sabotaging attitudes—such as believing that we are victims, powerless, fearful, doubting, unwilling to forgive, and so on—cut us off from the power and inherent worth of our true self. This denial of the truth of our beings is the spiritual cause of cancer and other diseases.

Disease is a message that there are psychological and spiritual issues that need to be healed. We are being given feedback that we are denying our true self or *spiritual self of pure love* and blocking our health and happiness.

PNI established a mind/body connection to illness and health. My studies and experience have shown me that there *is* a mind/body/spirit connection between disease and its reversal. *The cause of disease is psychological and spiritual, not physical.* Both need to be healed for the body to fully recover.

Ancient healing practices have shown me that *healing happens on the spiritual level*. Unless the spiritual cause of cancer is healed as well as the psychological cause, it will just keep coming back—sometimes in a different part of the body. Once we heal the psychological and spiritual cause, the energy blockages are released, and the body can heal itself.

As a psychologist and three-time cancer survivor, it is my experience that we can heal our bodies by changing the toxic attitudes that have disconnected us from the love of our true self. Because all healing happens on the spiritual level, we need to reconnect with this love, which is the most powerful healing energy there is. Then this love that is within us flows throughout the body, creating health and we are healed.

Marianne Williamson said in her book, *A Return to Love*:

> "Love is what we were born with. Fear is what we learn. The spiritual journey is the unlearning of fear and the acceptance of love back into our hearts."

When we feel lack of love, we feel fear. Fear takes many forms, such as anger, resentment, jealousy, anxiety, worry, doubt, hatred, shame, blame, judgment, unworthiness, and so on. Love opens the energy channels for the life force to flow smoothly, which enables the systems of the body to function harmoniously.

Fear and painful emotions produce the fight or flight response, which puts stress on the adrenal glands and the nervous system so that hormonal imbalances occur. Lack of love and emotional pain create a constant interruption of the healthy flow of the body systems—the cardiovascular, respiratory, endocrine, circulatory, digestive, nervous, eliminatory, and so on. These interruptions cause chemical imbalances that break the body down until the cells develop abnormal cells that are called cancer or disease.

As our fears are healed, we find the love of our true self underneath— which not only makes us feel good, it strengthens our immune system and heals us. And in the process, we get in touch with our own truth, worth, and magnificence.

The gift of disease is that it takes us from the physical level where we usually operate, into the emotional, mental, and finally into the spiritual level, to reconnect with our own true self—the source of all lasting healing. In this way, disease can become a voyage of rediscovery of our self.

Marianne Williamson continues in her book, *A Return to Love*:

"Love is the essential reality and our purpose on earth. To be consciously aware of it, to experience love in ourselves and others, is the meaning of life."

As we reconnect with our true selves, our bodies relax, our minds become quiet, and we get in touch with feelings of love—love for our self, love for others, and love for a higher power. Using this mind/body/spirit connection, *we have the power to heal our bodies.* And to create a joyful life that will nurture us mind, body, and soul.

Symptoms of disease are critical messages from our true self urging us to wake up and get back on course so that our bodies can once again be nourished by the love and joy within us that is always waiting to be felt. *Joy strengthens and rebuilds the immune system.* So it is important to follow our joy if we want to reverse or prevent cancer and other diseases.

I feel the healthiest when I am in my highest joy, and when I follow my own inner knowing. I find that taking nothing from the outside works best for me. I have all my needs taken care of from the inside. Physicians such as Deepak Chopra tell us that all the medicines we need are inside our body. When I am in joy, my body is able to manufacture all the vitamins and medicines I need, and the life-force energy within me supplies the energy that I need. When I am centered in that knowing, my life flows best, and I am in radiant health.

By following our joy, anything being held in the body that would block our health is brought to our awareness so we can release it—without harming ourselves or anyone else. In this way, our bodies become self-healing.

For example, I remember waking up one morning with a cold, feeling weak and miserable. "Cancer is probably back," was my first fearful thought. "I ate bad turkey yesterday; I should go back to eating organic food," was my next thought. "I should start taking vitamin C," quickly followed. "Wait a moment," I finally interjected, "you are *not* in your joy." Then I asked myself, "What will give you joy?"

The immediate response was "have some chocolate." I smiled and went out to get some chocolate—Nutrageous, that's my favorite. As I was eating the chocolate, I became aware of a deep anger I was holding onto, that I was not expressing or owning, but denying as ridiculous.

"Get into the anger, feel it. It's okay to feel angry," I encouraged myself.

Scenes from the past, from about 25 years ago, appeared in my mind's eye, incidents in which I felt hurt but did not know how to stand up for myself.

I started an inner dialogue with the people involved and said everything I felt in my heart. Then I allowed my anger full expression inside my head, telling that person who'd hurt me what a horrible thing it was to do to another human being.

I suddenly understood how frightened, insecure, and threatened that person was by my success, and I saw that she'd hurt me so she could build up her own image. As soon as I understood it, I felt compassion—and my cold disappeared instantly.

Dr. Margo de Kooker, in her article, "Psychoneuroimmunology," states:

> "Research in the field of mind/body medicine has revealed a collection of 'immune power' traits. These 'healthy habits' have stood up to the scrutiny of researchers, and individuals can develop them to serve as buffers against immune system breakdown and disease progression. They include being aware of your mind-body feedback; learning how to view life with a sense of commitment, control, and challenge; developing strengths to fall back on in the wake of loss and a capacity to confide traumas and feelings to yourself and others."

Part II will show you how to do just that.

When I finally stopped doing things that made me unhappy and began doing what brought me joy, I started feeling better. *Joy is the body's feedback that we are connected to our true self.* When we are truly happy, our bodies are healthy. Stop doing what makes you unhappy. Instead, follow your joy, do what energizes and revitalizes you and makes you feel alive!

I would ask myself, "What would bring me joy right now?" And then I would do it. I began to follow the path of the true self—our highest truth, that we are good, loving, worthwhile, and creative and know that we have something of intrinsic value to contribute to the world around us—and I discovered my heart's true bliss. This is my passion, my life's purpose.

Find your passion that brings you joy. This is what gives our life meaning and a reason to carry on. Envision living that passion and use your creative energies so that it can unfold. Refocus your mind off your disease to living your passion. This brings us back to life and to our true self, which rebuilds the immune system and creates healing.

Henry Dreher says in his book, *The Immune Power Personality*:

"Immune power is demonstrated in an individual who is able to find true joy and meaning, even health, when life offers up its most difficult challenges."

When I was first diagnosed with cancer after not paying attention to my body's signals to stop my stressful life, my body was really telling me, "Either you live the life that brings you joy, or I am checking out on you. Life is to be enjoyed, not burdened with *have to*s."

For clues to where you have not been paying attention to your body's signals, not listening to your own wisdom, denying your goodness and your needs, and making decisions against yourself, look in the areas where you have settled for what was expedient, rather than chosen your highest joy.

Here's a checklist of symptoms to show you how your body/mind/spirit systems communicate with you when you have settled for less than joy.

Symptoms Feedback Checklist

1. Physical Symptoms:
   - Lack of energy, lethargy, tiredness.
   - Pain.
   - Sickness.
   - Disease.

2. Emotional Symptoms:
   - Feeling bad, unhappy, stressed (fear, anxiety, depression, powerlessness, doubt, resentment)
   - Conflicted, unhappy relationships (anger, rage, yelling, victimhood).

3. Mental Symptoms:
   - Your thinking is negative, pessimistic, cynical and sarcastic.
   - Hypercritical, finding something wrong with everyone and everything. For example, "I'm better than you" way of thinking.
   - Putting down children, never seeing their good. For example, "You stupid, good for nothing, you will never amount to anything."

- Over-focusing on what's wrong with you, such as thinking "I'm not good enough."

4. Spiritual Symptoms:

   - Not inspired or hopeful about your future.

   - Lost your connection with your inherent love and goodness.

   - No passion for life. Lost your purpose. Life has no meaning.

   - Running after material things, prestige, and power, and feeling empty inside.

   - Lack of joy.

   - Disconnected from your spiritual source of inspiration, love, and joy.

Dr. O. Carl Simonton said, "Cancer is a message of love." Disease is urging us to correct our unhealthy attitudes, listen to our inner wisdom, and be our true self.

When I finally started to honor my true self and do the things that my heart craved, I began to follow my bliss. I noticed that magical miracles would unfold. I would meet new people, and synchronicity led me to wonderful new adventures. My life became so magnificent that I finally understood how my cancer was a message of love. It ended up being an incredible gift that changed my life radically. Most of my dreams have come true.

I remember often thinking, while I was living far away from the ocean that I loved, "I'm longing to live close to water, so why am I choosing to live here?" To live beside the ocean seemed like an impossible dream that only a few lucky or wealthy people could afford. It never occurred to me that a simple person like me could actually live at the beach. I now live by the ocean in Hawaii, and my life has unfolded in new, magical ways. If I can do it, so can you.

People with cancer and other diseases are dying miserable deaths because of ignorance and lack of knowledge. Doctors are doing the best they know how. However, all the deaths are unnecessary when there are better methods available—even though they may not yet be fully known or understood.

It will take some time to change the current approach to healing. Even when this knowledge is understood and accepted by traditional physicians, it will take years for the climate to change. New textbooks, new teachers, new thinking...it takes a long time for fresh ideas to be adopted. In the meantime, people are feeling tortured with pain and by treatments such as surgery and chemotherapy just as I was.

If I had waited until what I practiced was widely accepted by the traditional medical field before I gave these self-healing exercises a chance, it would have meant prolonging my torture—and inevitable death. Thank goodness I did not listen to authority figures who dictated to me that their knowing was more accurate than mine. I was terrified to listen to my own heart and challenge the traditional way of thinking that was all around me. But luckily for me, the terror of having to continue what to me felt like torture was greater than the fear of risking my life by taking it into my own hands.

I believe that disease is a solution to a larger problem. So many people today are overstressed, angry, jealous, and revengeful; they hurt one another in so many ways. People often lie, cheat, steal, manipulate, and harm each other. Even among the leaders of the country—in government, corporate, and religious organizations—crime is rampant. I believe that disease is the catalyst that the collective subconscious has found to force us to get back in touch with our goodness so we can live wholesome, worthwhile lives.

For example, when I wasn't voluntarily making changes in my life, cancer was the solution that my subconscious used to guide me back to my true self and to living a more joyful life. People are crying out to live joyful and meaningful lives. Their bodies are telling them, "Either you find a way to enjoy your life, or I am checking out on you," as my body told me.

The problems in our society are merely a reflection of the collective problems that dwell within each one of us. It is up to us to make changes within ourselves to feel more love, joy, peace, and health in our lives. If we want to enjoy living in a world that is a safe and healthy place to be, we need to begin healing ourselves. To me, the people challenging cancer and other diseases are the warriors who are ready to take on these diseases so that the world will wake up to its goodness.

The sobering statistic that cancer is the number-two killer in our society and soon predicted to be number one (replacing heart disease) is data that give us profound feedback. Because the deeper cause of heart disease is a closed heart and of cancer is a denial of the true self, these societal symptoms are mirroring back to us our collective longing to *connect with a higher self, a higher purpose, and a higher passion—enthusiasm and excitement about life.*

We need to become aware of how subconscious toxic decisions against ourselves rule and sabotage our lives. It's a self-destructive mechanism that can be changed, however. The first step is to make the changes in our emotional, mental and spiritual health. *The physical changes then follow the changes that are made inside. As the energies of peace, love, and joy are strengthened and grow to new levels of harmony, symptoms of pain, suffering, fear, and sickness begin to diminish.* Eventually there will be less and less sickness in people's lives. There will be no more need for it.

In Part II you will learn to read the messages your body is giving you so you can support the body's inherent healing process. You will discover how you denied your needs when you made decisions that acted against your true self of goodness and worthiness, and how to correct it. You will learn to listen to the doctor within and follow this guidance.

You will learn how to practice self-healing exercises to tap into the vital life force that energizes and heals the body. As pain and fear are relieved through the practice of these exercises, the body relaxes and the mind becomes quiet. Then you will learn to connect with your spiritual source, the source of all healing. Finally, you will learn to follow your heart's true bliss, the path of your true self.

These exercises redirect the mind back to the truth of your inherent goodness and worthiness, which sends signals to the brain to strengthen the immune system and begin the healing process. When these exercises are practiced regularly, cancer and other diseases begin to be reversed or prevented.

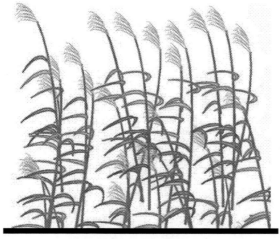

Part II

The 9 Steps Program to Reverse or Prevent Cancer and Other Diseases

Chapter 4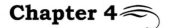

Step One: Making a Decision to Be Well

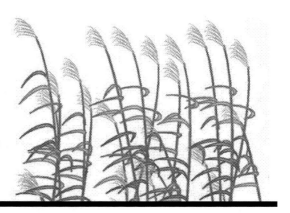

"Day before yesterday I was in the hospital and told that I only have a few days to live. The doctors said that my body is filled with the AIDS virus, and there is nothing they can do to help me." Edward, a workshop participant, continued, "I got up and left the hospital unnoticed and walked home. I heard you speak on the radio and your story moved me to come and see if your work can help me. It's amazing that I am even walking since there is a whole city of AIDS inside me."

"Illness has very little to do with what we *think* it is," I replied. "In my experience and understanding, diseases—including AIDS—develop because of a weakness in the mind/body/spirit system."

"What did you say?" asked Edward, leaning forward eagerly.

I continued to explain, "It's the degree to which we feel painful emotions and lack of self-love that often determines which illness will show up in our bodies."

Edward looked stunned.

"Sickness is just a feedback system," I replied. "In my opinion, the AIDS virus is a reflection of negative thought patterns, which can be identified and changed. Then the body has the ability to heal itself."

"I wish I could believe that," Edward said.

"It is up to you. You don't have to believe everything the doctors say if you don't want to. As often as possible, focus on your body as though it's already healed, and choose to believe in that image, instead of what the doctors told you."

Edward got quiet after that. Then, during the workshop, while practicing the visualization to heal disease, he remembered a scene from childhood where he'd felt humiliated.

"My father was an alcoholic and told me that I wasn't worth anything. His behavior was really destructive to my mother and me. I wanted to hate my father or call him stupid, but instead I hated myself for being worthless and powerless to stop him."

Edward discovered the subconscious decisions he had made: "I am worthless and powerless as I am. I don't deserve to exist, and I should die."

"I realize that these subconscious decisions have been sabotaging my health," he continued. "Now I can see that my father couldn't judge if I was worthy. I know if I want to heal, I have to forgive him and myself."

He changed from being victimized by old toxic attitudes to making a new healing decision, "I am fine as I am, and the more I allow myself to know that and to love myself just as I am, the more I feel that I deserve to live in good health."

Edward agreed to continue practicing healing his emotional wounds daily, to identify all the toxic attitudes that had caused his immune system to break down and then change those thoughts into healing decisions that create health. In addition, he agreed to practice the hypothalamic orgasmic response exercise daily to strengthen his immune system.

Two and a half years later, I received an e-mail from Edward, "My health is great....My T cells are almost above normal and my white blood cells are above normal. You should see me; you wouldn't even recognize me." A few months later, Edward called to report that his T cells were above normal.

In February 2003, Edward told me about his journey back to health, "When symptoms showed up, at first I fell back into old patterns of thinking and said to myself, 'Oh, here is the sickness again; I was just kidding myself.' My healing process brought me into deeper layers of my beliefs about doubting myself, which needed to shift gears into more certainty.

"From time to time, I would get conditions that strike weakened immune systems, such as shingles. At first, I would think what my doctors think: that I am still sick, and what I'm doing is not working. I started doubting that

I healed myself. Then as I worked on healing the deeply rooted toxic decisions, the symptoms got better rapidly. My doctors know that it takes about five weeks for shingles to heal. They were surprised when I healed them in four days. They knew that I hadn't filled the prescriptions they gave me. So they were curious to find out what I was doing."

"What was their response?" I asked Edward.

"First they tried to discount it. But some doctors were intrigued with how I was able to change my blood. My T cells are still above normal. One doctor told me I have the blood of a 25-year old, and I am 38."

The Complete Program to Reverse Disease

In Part II, I will explore the complete program that allowed me to reverse my own cancer and helped my clients and students around the world to heal or prevent disease.

In addition to a Daily Healing Routine, there are exercises to relieve pain, shrink tumors, strengthen the immune system, and heal disease. There are exercises to improve your ability to visualize, quiet the mind, and release tiredness. You will find exercises to heal your unhealthy attitudes and emotional pain as well as to turn your doubt into certainty that you can be healed. And there are exercises to learn how to use spiritual energy to enhance your healing. Finally, you will find exercises to help you follow your heart's bliss, discover your passion, make better choices, and manifest the healthy, happy life you were born to live.

Also included is the self-healing exercise that Jack Canfield, cocreator of *Chicken Soup for the Soul* series, called "The Five-Minute Cure."

The first step in the program to reverse or prevent disease is to make the decision to be well. Until that decision is made, the body remains in a state of continual breakdown. Once that decision is made, a new healthy message is sent to the brain, filling the body with hope and joy, which then releases healing chemicals and hormones.

To regain your health, it is essential to make a decision to be in radiant health. It is important to persuade the mind to adopt healthy healing perceptions that produce wellness images in the brain, which then "out-picture" in the body as health. As you proceed through this program, you will be carefully shown how to create healing images so that instead of seeing yourself as diseased with cancer or another illness, you will see yourself as being well.

You will look inside at the decisions that have not served you and make new decisions that can create health. For example, you don't have to believe what others have told you if you don't want to. It's your choice. *You have the power within you to decide to choose the attitudes, beliefs, thoughts, perceptions, and images that you wish to nurture and allow to grow.* You don't have to believe that you have a disease if you don't want to.

Ask yourself, "Do you want to believe in pain and sickness?" Wait for an honest answer. If it's "no," then tell yourself, "I don't have to believe anything I don't want to." You may hear your mind respond, "But I'll be fooling myself; the doctors say I am dying of cancer." *Do you want to believe you are dying of cancer, knowing that that attitude alone can kill you?* If the answer is "no," then continue repeating, "I don't have to if I don't want to." Keep on doing it until you hear and feel a relief inside.

By now you're asking, "You mean I don't have to believe the doctors?"

Do you want to? If your inner response is, "No, I don't want to, but I have no choice. I have to believe what the doctors say," consider this: Suppose the doctors are wrong. There is a chance that they don't know. Doctors have been found to be wrong on many occasions before. They are fallible human beings like everyone else—no more, no less. You may hear a response, "I suppose they could be wrong, although it is very unlikely. The X-rays and biopsies show cancer."

Now I want you to pay full attention to what I'm going to say next. *If cancer is just a feedback mechanism telling you what your thoughts have caused, all you have to do is change the unhealthy thoughts that caused the cancer to begin with to healthy thoughts—and the cancer will disappear!*

The body is neutral. It cannot be manipulated to reflect something other than what you believe inside. Your body does not care. It's like a computer. Put different thoughts in your body's computer. Make a decision to believe those thoughts free of any shadow of doubt. Be certain in your new decisions. Convince your mind to believe your new thoughts. And don't allow any doubts to interfere—yours or others—including your doctors.

A client once said to me, "When I read articles or watch television shows that talk about statistics and convincingly show how there is no cure for cancer, I feel terribly sick, frightened, and disheartened. Doubts come in and people's opinions that this positive thinking is all rubbish suddenly become my reality."

What can you do to protect yourself from being influenced by negativity? Give yourself permission to stop reading articles that upset you and to stop watching television shows or movies that make you doubt yourself. No one has complete knowledge of everything. No one can be that arrogant to insist that they have all the answers. Some answers, yes; but there is so much more that has not yet been discovered.

It is important to understand that there is a lot of knowledge that we can open up to before it is scientifically proven and widely accepted. Before Christopher Columbus discovered America, it was widely accepted that the world was flat. Columbus's discovery did not make the world round, it just expanded people's perception so they could accept the truth that was there all along.

As I mentioned in Part I, the latest research in PNI indicates that it is our negative or toxic attitudes that make us sick and eventually kill us. The effect of strong sarcastic, skeptical, negative attitudes on the body is sickness. If these destructive attitudes are not changed, the discomfort grows and the sickness gets worse.

The good news is that attitudes are easy to change. They can be changed by the mere decision to be open to experimenting with new ways of thinking. What do you have to lose? Let the negative attitudes within you die along with the disease and you will stay alive. Let your body regain its health and let your life be treasured as a precious gift so that you can live your life in joy.

In this program, you will learn to entertain attitudes that support only the highest in you—your goodness, worthiness, and health. *Experience has shown me that attitude alone can heal.* Therefore, to facilitate your healing, you will be shown how to hold only healthy, healing attitudes about yourself and your body.

And you will look deeper at your long-held negative attitudes that have caused your health to break down in the first place. Finally, you will learn how to easily change them.

Let's begin with an exercise to help you make a decision to be well. My students have received great benefit from this exercise. One of my students, Marlene, a physical exercise teacher from New Brunswick, N.J., who was challenging a terminal disease, had this to say:

> "I feel very grateful for this exercise, which I believe has not only helped me make new decisions to heal rather than give up and die,

but has also helped me change my life. I always made fun of this stuff as crazy until I tried it out, thinking that I have nothing to lose, so I gave it a chance. Well, I am overwhelmed at how easy and wonderful it is to make new decisions. Before, I didn't feel good inside. I felt quite miserable, but didn't want anyone to know it. I was too proud to admit it, but it feels so good to no longer be enslaved to that way of thinking. I am free and *my disease is gone for good.* I now know it was a blessing in disguise."

Exercise to Make a Decision to Be Well

To make a decision to be well, follow these four steps:

1. Think of an attitude that makes you feel unhappy. For example, an attitude that would make you feel unhappy, which I have found to create disease, is: "I am not lovable as I am." This is a common issue for those challenging cancer.

2. Now make a new decision to love and support yourself, then practice it, saying: "I am lovable as I am. I am okay. I am fine just the way I am, and I decide to choose to love all aspects of me, my strengths and my weaknesses. I make a decision to live; I deserve to have a life."

One reason we don't love ourselves is because we buy into others' beliefs about us. I remember as a child deciding that I must believe others' thoughts and criticism of me. Even though deep inside, I knew it was not true, I was afraid that if I didn't act and show that I believed what they said, they would not love me. Later on in life, I continued believing lies, and my inner conflict was: "If I am successful, others will suffer the pain of jealousy and will find ways to attack and hurt me. I have to buy into their beliefs even if they are against me." *I then acted against myself in order to be loved. When you act against yourself, disease shows up as the physical expression of your destructive inner thoughts.*

The body is a feedback system. It gives us warnings: "These are the thoughts you are holding onto. They are killing you. Stop acting against yourself."

3. Think of a decision you've made that has created conflict within you. Exaggerate it, open it up as fully as you can, imagine it

engulfing your whole body, the whole room you are in. Now love it; flood it with love. Imagine the love is the size of the world. Now surrender it to a higher power, to God, to the universe, to Mother Earth, to the ocean or to the trees as fertilizer, as pure love to nurture and nourish all.

4.   Make a new decision that you are well, feeling loved and lovable. Here are some attitudes you may wish to adopt. Repeat them sincerely as you envision your life filled with blessings.

   ◆ The more I believe that I can get well and heal, the more I heal.

   ◆ The more I allow myself to love myself, the more love I feel inside. The more love I feel inside, the more I love others. The more I love others, the more others love themselves. The more others love themselves, the more they love me.

   ◆ The more decisions I make to enjoy every minute of my life, the more fun life becomes and the healthier I get.

   ◆ The more I sincerely practice these new decisions, the more my health improves.

   ◆ My new decisions are stronger than the old toxic decisions.

   ◆ The more I focus on my new decisions, the stronger they grow.

   ◆ One year from now, I will be celebrating life in radiant health with wonderful people, enjoying the work that fulfills my dreams. I look forward to all of life's exciting adventures that will come my way. I am willing to feel these feelings of celebration right now. Why wait? The more I feel them now, the faster they show up in my life.

Effortlessly feel these new thoughts vibrating in every cell of your body. Feel them, touch them, smell them, hear them, taste them while repeating the new decisions over and over inside, seeing yourself already healed, living a full, enjoyable life.

Chapter 5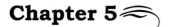

Step Two: Healing Your Emotional Pain

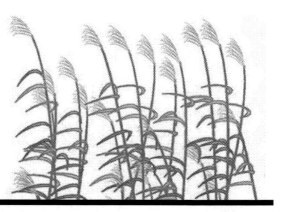

"I have had migraine headaches for years. I've tried everything from conventional medicine to alternative therapies and nothing helped," said Elsa, a brilliant businesswoman who built a million-dollar company from scratch.

At a seminar in San Francisco, she shared her story about being constantly criticized since childhood by her mother. "The message I received every day until I left home at 16 was, 'What's the matter with you? When will you grow up? You are a stupid, ugly, good-for-nothing idiot. You will never amount to anything.'"

During the exercise to heal emotional pain, Elsa had an inner dialogue with her mother and began to express the emotions that had long been held inside. She started to release the hatred she felt for her mother when she recognized that it was poisoning her body. She formed a new healing decision, "I am lovable and good enough as I am."

After practicing the exercise several times a day, Elsa reported that it was the first time in years that she woke up in the morning without pain.

Because Elsa was not yet ready to forgive her mother, I suggested that she continue practicing the exercises at home. A year later, she reported that she was able to release the toxic feelings of anger and hatred, transmuting them into forgiveness and love. "I first forgave myself for giving my power away and blocking my joy by believing my mother's harsh words. I then forgave my mother for not knowing how she was hurting me."

Elsa's migraines had diminished, but they would come back as soon as she felt overstressed and stopped practicing her healing exercises. She thought she had forgiven her mother completely, but discovered that she did not want to have any contact with her. "As soon as I speak with my mother on the phone, I start feeling miserable again."

I suggested that she take time out of her busy schedule to slow down and be quiet, simplify her life, and make practicing the healing exercises a priority until the migraines disappear completely, and she feels strong and centered within her power.

Later, Elsa told me that her migraines had disappeared completely. "Taking time out to be quiet and practice the exercise to heal emotional pain as well as performing the daily healing routine three times a day has made the difference," she reported. "I have been listening to your tapes of the exercises daily, which made it easier for me to relax and follow the instructions effortlessly."

Not only did Elsa reverse her painful headaches, but she began to enjoy her life. New creativity emerged and she started painting, which gives her great joy.

Emotional pain is one of the biggest blocks to creating health. Extensive mind/body research has shown that unresolved emotions are the basis for disease. So the second step is to release the emotional pain that not only makes you feel bad, but keeps the toxic attitudes in place that is causing your disease. As you feel and release all the energy in the body that makes you feel bad, major healing occurs. In the process, the decisions and attitudes that caused the emotional pain are identified and can then be changed.

From my experience working with people with cancer and other diseases, I notice that there is a disease-prone personality and that people with this personality have one thing in common—they do not feel deeply loved or lovable, which causes feelings of insecurity. Anxiety, fear, and self-blame are then the emotions that are experienced instead of the secure feelings of love. Fear and anxiety trigger the body's fight or flight response, which release chemicals that overtax the immune system, weakening its ability to function effectively, resulting in disease.

Feelings of self-hatred or lack of love are usually learned in childhood from parents, teachers, family, and friends who don't know how to feel or express love. We have generations of dysfunctional parenting to understand and heal.

When I first started working as a psychologist and witnessed my clients' emotional pain because of their parents' inability to love them, I became acutely aware of my own emotional pain. I realized that the pain I was feeling was because my father had never told me that he loved me. I was living in New Jersey at the time, and I decided to visit my parents in Israel with the intention of healing this issue.

I resolved to be courageous and tell my father that I loved him. I was amazed at how difficult it was to do.

Finally, I gathered my courage, saying, "I want you to know that I love you, Daddy."

He looked shocked and embarrassed. All he could do in return was make a feeble jest: "But I hate you."

I felt anger well up within me. I had a desire to curse at him and walk away. Instead, I was wise enough to understand that he couldn't help it; he was too confused and did not know how to respond with what he truly felt. "That's okay, you don't have to love me; I can still love you," I responded, smiling. His face melted, and he invited me to go out to lunch with him. That was the first time he had ever invited me out.

As I was leaving to come back to the United States, my mother nudged him and said, "Tell her that you love her."

He couldn't do it.

Just as I was walking out the door, I heard him yell out, "I love you."

At a later time, my father explained to me that no one had ever told him that they loved him. His parents never told him, and he did not know what love was.

"What is love?" he asked me. I did not know how to explain it to him then. He has since passed away.

Had I known then what I know now, I would say:

"Love is caring about you so much that I would never hurt you. It means I will always be there to support you and to understand you so fully that you don't shut yourself down, so you blossom to your full potential. I admire the gifts you have, the good qualities and strength you possess. When I think of you, I feel a sensation of warmth and joy vibrating inside my heart. I feel a connection, an intimate knowing of who you really are. I want to soothe your pain away, to help you heal any pain or suffering you have had to put up with in your life."

As I was focusing on my father's image, I felt a warmth in my heart for him that I had not felt before. I felt as though a part of my heart that still was not fully open to feeling my love for him because of the hurtful things that he said and did, finally opened. As I focused on the pain he had to put up with in his life, I saw him releasing his pain through tears of healing. Even though my father had already left his body, it felt as if he were able to release this block through my loving understanding. And his love for himself and my love for myself increased.

Imagine your own parents are in front of you. It does not matter if they are dead or alive. Say the loving things to your parents you wish you could have expressed and notice how it feels inside your heart. I also recommend the practice of telling your parents, family, and friends—face to face or in your imagination as much as possible—what love is, especially at times when you feel emotionally moody or drained.

Healing images of forgiveness not only make you feel good, they also create health. The faster your heart opens to feeling emotions of love, compassion, and understanding, the faster you heal. The brain releases chemicals and hormones that respond to these images of love and convey this message to the rest of the body. Messages of calm, peace, joy, love, safety, protection, comfort, and pleasure are transmitted through the blood to every cell. The immune system is strengthened, and the natural healing mechanisms take over, creating health.

Exercise to Heal Emotional Pain

To heal your emotional pain, complete the following 12 steps:

1. Feel the emotion you are experiencing right now. Whether it is fear, anger, guilt, jealousy, shame, blame, sadness, grief, loss, depression, or failure, feel it.

2.　Close your eyes and describe the sensations you are noticing or feeling. Closing your eyes makes it easier to focus inside and feel your sensations fully. Say: "Now I am feeling _____" and fill in the blank. For example: "Now I am noticing the room I am in. Now I am feeling my hands. Now I am feeling my closed eyes. Now I am feeling the sensations in my chest. Now I am feeling the sensations in my heart. Now I am feeling pain in my heart. Now I am feeling tightness in my neck. Now I am feeling my legs shaking. Now I am noticing a memory passing by. Now I am feeling my emotional pain."

3.　Describe the pain as vividly as you can. For example, "I feel a burning sensation in my spine, pressure in my abdomen, fearful sensation in my whole body, sharp pain in my thigh," or whatever you feel.

4.　Move into the emotional pain and give it a voice. Let it express itself fully as though it were a person within you. This person may say, "I feel _____" and fill in the gap. For example: "I feel sorry for myself. I have been treated unfairly, misunderstood, trampled upon, ridiculed, crushed, disrespected, unloved, and uncared for."

5a.　Have a dialogue with that person inside you. Respond by saying whatever comes up in your mind. Don't worry whether it makes sense or not. For example, you may say: "Who made you feel this way?" Response: "You are making me feel this way the most. You believe what others think or say instead of loving me and comforting me."

5b.　Keep the dialogue going back and forth. You may respond by saying: "Tell me all you feel. I am here to listen and help you, to comfort and love you." A response may be, "I feel hopeless, helpless, angry, and frustrated."

6.　Respond by feeling your anger (or whatever emotion you are feeling) fully. Express it. Take a pillow and beat the pillow up, pretending it represents the people you are angry with. Give yourself time to experience the energy of anger as fully as possible. It sometimes takes as long as an hour or several hours to allow the energy to flow.

7. Now move to the feelings beneath the anger: the hurt and the powerlessness. Breathe and relax into the sensation of powerlessness. Allow yourself to cry for as long as you need to. Be with it, own it, embrace it. Allow it to be felt as totally as possible. Breathe in and out of the emotional pain as though you are massaging it, creating space in the center of the pain.

8. Now imagine the first time you felt that pain. What happened? Recreate that scene as if it were happening right now in the present. For example, you might have first felt the pain of depression when you were a little child and someone criticized or yelled at you, or your parents began arguing or fighting in front of you.

9a. Have a dialogue with your parents as if they were right there right now. Place two chairs in front of you, and imagine them sitting there listening to you intently. Be the little child and tell them everything you are feeling inside. For example: "When you argue, I feel frightened that I did something wrong, that it is my fault, that you will hurt each other and I will be abandoned. I feel that you don't love me, and that I am unlovable." Continue telling them everything you are feeling inside.

9b. Now, be your parents and respond. For example, they may say in their ignorance, "Shut up! Children must be seen and not heard," or something equally harsh.

9c. Respond to that, and say whatever it takes to shake them up enough to tell the real truth.

9d. Again, be your parents and respond on a deeper level. For example, they may then say something like: "We are too proud to admit that we are horrible bullies, that we are cowards, that we pick on you because you are less powerful then us, that we think so little about ourselves, that we are so afraid of life and having to face the hardships of survival. It is not your fault; it is our stupidity. We are truly sorry for hurting you. We don't know how to give you the love you deserve and the caring we wish we knew how to share. Please forgive us. We love you very much whether we can show it or not and whether you know it or not; we are just ignorant.

9e.   Imagine them taking you in their arms and hugging you while you all cry together.

9f.   Imagine how hurt they felt in their childhood and how afraid they were of their parents. Their parents believed in what society believed, that "to spare the rod spoils the child" is the right approach to child rearing. Imagine them being more hurt than you were and not knowing how to react.

9g.   Tell them what you need from them in order to heal and forgive. For example: "I need you to tell me that you love me, that you are happy I am your child. Tell me how wonderful I am, how special and important. Tell me what my strengths are and that you will always protect me and be there for me."

9h.   Breathe in deeply and open your heart to receive their love. Remember, the brain does not care whether the images are real or imagined. The brain releases chemicals and hormones according to the images you visualize.

9i.   Create healing images of sharing deep, meaningful love with one another. Imagine your parents saying to you all that you yearned to hear as a child. Know that if they'd known how to say it, they would have loved to have done so. They want you to be happy, well adjusted, productive, healthy, and a successful member of society.

10.   You can now be the perfect parent to yourself. Take another pillow and hug it, imagine that it is you when you were young. Tell the little child all that you would want him or her to hear. "I love you. I will be loyal to you from now

on. I will not abandon you by believing what others say about you. I will protect you with my love." Continue saying everything in your heart to make the child that is you feel loved, protected, and whole.

11.   Be the little child and feel all that love pouring into your little body. Make new decisions to heal the emotional pain that has accumulated over the years. "I now decide to know that I am lovable, good, admired, respected, and acknowledged. The more I love and approve of myself, the more others love and approve of me, and it grows. I can do it; I can feel good; I deserve it." Keep on hugging the little child that is you until you feel so good that you want to get up and go outside to play. See yourself laughing playfully.

12.   Now open your eyes and describe the sensations you are feeling. Say: "Now I am feeling _____" and fill in the blank. Do this until you are totally present and feeling good. For example: "Now I am feeling my chest being open and free. Now I am feeling my face smiling. Now I am feeling good inside." And so on.

Because emotional pain is one of the biggest blocks to creating health, I recommend you practice this exercise every day or every other day until you feel relief. Then do it once a week and, finally, once a month until the pain is completely healed.

In addition, here's a quick exercise to help melt those blocks.

Quick Emotional Healing Exercise

Usually emotional pain is stored in the heart, which is the place where we feel our heartaches and where we tend to be very harsh on ourselves.

To help melt emotional blocks, complete the following three steps:

1.   Imagine whenever you remember, that your heart is like the sun, radiating love and warmth throughout your body and toward everyone and everything in all directions.

2.   While you are beaming these rays of light, say, "I love you," and "be healed."

3.   Breathe this light in and out of your heart all day and all night long, whenever it occurs to you to do it. Soon it will become second nature.

Chapter 6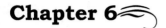

Step Three: Healing Your Toxic Attitudes

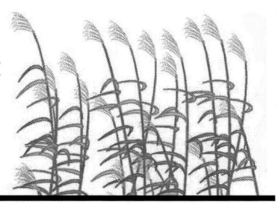

Alice was afraid of a recurrence of breast cancer after surgery and chemotherapy. When she attended a workshop, she resisted believing in her own power to heal herself and stay well. When I mentioned that it is our choice to stop suffering and feel good, her immediate response was, "I find that hard to believe."

"If that's your attitude, that's what will happen in your life," I said. "You will keep on making it hard to believe that you can feel good inside."

During the workshop, Alice learned how to change her unhealthy attitudes into new healing decisions, such as, "The more I love and nurture my ability to feel good inside, the better I feel."

A year later, Alice reported doing well until some of the women in the cancer support group she was attending passed away after their cancer spread. Their deaths triggered her fears of a recurrence.

After taking a refresher workshop, Alice practiced the exercise to heal toxic attitudes and chose new healing decisions on a daily basis, and she reported, "This exercise has strengthened me in surprising ways. When my yoga teacher had a recurrence of breast cancer, she said to me, 'You will have a recurrence too—it's only a matter of time.' I instantly responded, 'If you can't see me as healthy and cancer-free forever, then I am going to have to stay away from you.' I would never have been able to stand up for myself like that before.

Your exercise has not only helped me prevent a recurrence, it has helped me develop the inner strength to not take on the toxic beliefs of others."

Step three involves healing your toxic attitudes that cause disease. It is important to know that every decision you make has a quantifiable health value. As you understand the health value of your decisions, you can make healing changes. Let's start by measuring the health value of your attitudes.

Measuring the Health Value of an Attitude

We rarely think of the attitudes upon which we build our lives as having a health value. However, not knowing the effect our attitudes have on our health can kill us. Dr. Robert Maultsby of Howard University has developed a scale that measures the health value of an attitude or belief. I have found this scale to be very helpful.

Dr. O. Carl Simonton was the first one to bring this scale to my attention more than a decade ago. The scale is based on five questions:

1. Does this belief make me feel the way I wish to feel?
2. Does it help protect my health and my life?
3. Does it help me achieve my short- and long-term goals in life?
4. Does it help me resolve my most undesirable conflict?
5. Is it based on fact?

Test each of your attitudes with this scale. If the answer to two or three out of the five questions is "no," then it is an unhealthy attitude. If you continue believing it, it will affect your health.

A question I am frequently asked is, how do I develop trust and faith in my ability to heal myself? Trust is an attitude, a resting of the mind in the confidence that you will heal your body. Faith is also an attitude. It is a profound level of trust, a profound resting of the mind by having absolute confidence in your body being healed. It is your choice in which attitudes you wish to place your confidence. It is up to you whether you choose healing attitudes that nurture and build your trust and faith in your body's ability to create radiant health.

Finding the Toxic Attitudes That Caused Disease

For many years, I saw hundreds of clients at my Biofeedback, Psychology, and Stress Management Center in New Jersey. My expertise was in helping alleviate psychosomatic disorders, such as hypertension, ulcers, rheumatism, arthritis, back pain, all forms of physical pain, cold hands and feet, insomnia, headaches, migraines, phobias, anxiety, depression, and other mind/body discomforts and diseases.

Having attended biofeedback conferences and seminars on a regular basis, it became clear to me how the mind affects the body. Numerous studies indicated the ability to reverse physiological disorders with the mind. I understood, as I mentioned earlier, that there is a physiological response in every cell of the body to every thought we think.

When I placed the sensors of the GSR (galvanic skin response) biofeedback instrument on a client's fingertips, both the client and I were able to notice the physiological changes occurring as we listened to the changes in the feedback tones.

For example, when a client started talking about her relationship with her mother, the pitch of the tone would increase rapidly, indicating a rise in her body's level of stress. When I would introduce pleasant scenes, such as a beautiful beach for her to focus on, the sound would decrease to a quiet tone. We noticed that as soon as she thought about her mother, her stress level would rise. I would then use Gestalt dialogues with her to clarify how her attitudes about her mother affected her and her body. She was able to identity the toxic decisions she had made and change them so that she could bring that relationship into healthy interaction.

Making New Healing Decisions

Changing hidden self-sabotaging decisions has been a profound tool in showing me how to reverse disease. When we identify and change toxic decisions to healing decisions, positive changes take place. As the old destructive attitudes change into constructive perceptions, the body's diseases diminish and disappear. Feelings of well-being and an optimistic view of life are enlivened.

It is important for you to find the toxic decision that you made that caused your cancer or other disease so you can heal it. Until you do that, the disease can return—sometimes in a different place.

For example, as I shared in Part I, after having my left breast removed, the cancer came back two more times—in different places in my right breast—until I tracked the cause to the core toxic decision that kept the cancer reoccurring. Neither surgery nor chemotherapy could stop it. The cancer kept returning until I healed the core toxic decision I made when I was a small child.

When challenging cancer, I discovered the following exercise to be an important part of the healing process so that internal changes can then occur.

Exercise to Heal Toxic Attitudes and Choose New Healing Decisions

It is good to do this exercise when you are emotionally upset, usually at night when the deeper emotions are felt.

To heal unhealthy attitudes and make new healing decisions, complete the following steps:

1. First identify the root decisions that made you sick. One of the best ways to do this is to delve deep within whatever pain you feel. Experience that pain as fully as possible; exaggerate it, make it worse in order to identify the core decision.

2. Breathe into the depth of the emotional or physical pain and develop an internal dialogue. For example, you may address your heart saying, "Tell me what you are feeling. I really want to know. I am listening." Then wait for your heart to respond. You may hear nothing at first. Ask again more sincerely. Open yourself to connect with your heart's sensations. Usually past wounds, from when you were criticized, put down, hurt, humiliated, abandoned, or rejected are stored in the heart. Listen with an open mind and a willingness not to judge or ridicule yourself. Scenes from the past will pass through your mind.

3. Open these pictures and imagine living those events right now. For example, imagine the time in your life when you

experienced the most pain, when your parents, teachers, or friends were mean to you. Now be that age right now, and imagine they are in front of you.

4. Tell them the whole truth. Know that you are safe now and it is fine to expose everything to them. You may be 5 years old, but you possess the wisdom of a mature person.

A dialogue may be as follows:

"I feel _____." Always start with how you truly feel. "I feel so small when you make fun of me. I feel that you don't care about me and want to hurt me. All you care about is yourself. You try to impress your friends by putting me down. I feel hurt, alone, abandoned, worthless, unlovable, ugly..." or whatever you were feeling at the time.

Allow yourself to say anything that comes up during the exercise. You may start crying as the words spill out, but allow whatever happens to happen. You may feel angry. Take a pillow and beat it with your hands, expressing your anger out loud. Let it all out as fully as possible. Take as much time as needed to do this. Some people are able to feel a release in a few minutes; it may take others a few hours.

5. Next, imagine that person or persons you blame responding to you with honesty. They may say something like: "I was stupid, I didn't know what I was doing, I had no idea it would be so hurtful to you. The fun I made of you was only a reflection of how I was feeling inside about myself. I hated myself, feeling that I was not good enough, and I dumped this stress on you. I am truly sorry for the horrible things I said and did to you. I wouldn't blame you if you never forgave me, though I do ask your forgiveness. I don't want you to suffer; I want you feel good and be successful in all areas of your life..." and so on. Say whatever your imagination leads you to say.

Often, clients tell me, "My parents will never apologize like that, they are too proud." My response is, "They would love to be able to express the truth if they only knew how liberating it would be to them and to you; they are just not aware."

6.   Continue with the dialogue for as long as it takes to release all that you have been holding onto inside. You may wish to write it down in a journal or record it on a tape. Do this process with the many emotions that you may be experiencing in your life, be it guilt, jealousy, resentment, anger, frustration, irritation, hatred, shame, blame, sadness, fear, or any other emotion.

7.   Now, identify the decision you made about yourself because of the incidents in your imaginary dialogue. For example, "I must make fun of myself and treat myself with disrespect if others treat me that way." Or, "I have to feel bad inside when others behave in ways that hurt me." Or, "There is something wrong with me. I am flawed and not worth taking care of."

8.   Now, identify the decision you made about life. For example, "Life is difficult; it's a struggle to survive. I will never amount to anything." Or, "You have to feel pain in life."

9.   Now, identify the decision you made about other people. For example, "Other people are more important than me—they are wiser, stronger, and wealthier, and they know more and are better than me." Or, "People are mean, and I must stay alone in order to survive."

10. Write down your toxic decisions in your journal.

11. Now, continue the dialogue with the scenes you were working with, and tell them what you need from them in order to heal. You may wish to ask for what you needed from them as a child or at any time during your life. For example: "What I need from you, Dad, is to tell me how much you love me, how proud you are of me, and how much joy I bring into your life. That you will always be there for me to support me, to stand behind me, to guide me, to protect me, to make me feel safe and wanted."

12.   Now imagine taking that child in your arms. Take a pillow and imagine that it's you when you were that child. Hug yourself, and talk from the heart to the child that was you. Be the perfect father, mother, teacher, brother, sister, or friend to the child.

You may say something like, "You are wonderful, you are good just as you are; you are okay. People were too stressed out; they couldn't help it. You can feel good inside no matter what people say or do on the outside. You are in charge of your thoughts and your feelings. I love you, I will be loyal to you, I will not hurt you, I will not abandon you..." and so on.

Feel the love pouring in and out of your heart. Say things that make you feel that love. Ask the child that was you or your heart if there is something it longs to do. Explore the possibility of opening your heart very deeply. Great secrets are stored in the heart. You may wish to say, "Today my beloved, I open myself to you to receive your love." Love is the most healing energy there is. Open to that love, deepen it, and immerse yourself in it as fully and totally as possible.

13.   Spend an hour a day placing your hands on your chest connecting with that energy of love. You may do it last thing at night, when you wake up during the night, or first thing in the morning. Imagine washing your heart with the water of your love or God's love.

For some people, it works better to feel God's love washing away the past. For other people, just repeating the name of God cleanses the heart and soul each time they remember and repeat the name. They report experiencing an energy of holiness that lives in the garden of the soul.

If God is love and love is God, then seeing love everywhere in each person you meet and in every place you go, you connect with the source of love. In this way you realize that there is no difference between you, love, God, or them. If love is inside you and you live with that love all the time, you become the embodiment of love. As you invoke the light of love for your healing, you move to a new path, a new way. Mentally see your life healed, your body healed. Open your mind and heart as wide as you can to feel the love flowing through you that brings the healing.

14.   Make a decision to heal.

15. Now you are ready to make new healing decisions and empower them with your love. Take out the paper on which you wrote down your decisions, and change each one to its opposite. For example, if the old decision was, "I must feel miserable if people don't respect me or if I don't get what I want out of life," a healing decision would be, "The more I choose to respect myself and feel good inside, no matter what happens outside, the better I feel. And the better I feel, the more clarity I have to act in ways that serve me."

It's important that your mind believes in your new decision. If there is resistance, you may wish to take small steps. For example, "I am lovable just as I am" may seem unreal to you. You may not feel it yet, and your mind will reject that decision subconsciously. You may wish to start with, "The more I open to loving myself just as I am, the more lovable I feel. The more lovable I feel, the more lovable I become. The more I love myself, the more lovable I am. The more I feel and focus on this love, the more it grows and the healthier and happier I become."

16. Connect to life in the way you wish to feel. Make a decision to feel good inside. When you are successful in feeling joyful and fulfilled with a sense of satisfaction for one whole day, you will notice physical changes in your body. You will experience less pain, more love, and more peace. When you are able to feel these good feelings a few days in a row, you will notice how your body gradually regains health.

17. Make a conscious decision to choose to be your true self, which is passionate and enthusiastic about life. Remember when you made important decisions in your life, how you pondered over and over in your mind about the value of your decisions? Step out of your history, your past, and imagine this moment to be your new history, the way you want to be and feel.

Remind yourself that once you choose consciously, there is no need to go back to old ways of thinking. Be clear that the new decision is good for you and will help you regain health, strength, creativity, and productivity. A natural by-product will be success in all circumstances of your life.

18. Focus on how the natural healing mechanisms of the body are activated. Focus on the wisdom of your body that knows how to heal itself. Keep the body in a calm, tranquil, happy state for as long as possible. This is important because the feelings of love, trust, joy, and peace are the *fuel* that strengthens the immune system.

Practicing your new decisions three times a day for 10 to 20 minutes after deep relaxation or meditation will produce the best results. It usually takes around two months with regular, sincere practice for the new decision to penetrate the subconscious, and grow from seed to fruit. As soon as the new decision penetrates the subconscious, you will notice that you start living your life according to your new choices. As you practice repeating your decisions in a fresh new way, they blossom. Your new thoughts start powerfully affecting your life in direct proportion to the trust you place in them.

19. Cultivate confidence and trust in the decisions of your choice. Nurture them, nourish them with love, bless them, and see them grow, as you water the seeds. *They listen and absorb the nourishment you feed them with every word you utter and every thought you think.* They blossom best with the nourishing words of love, joy, peace, harmony, and passion for life.

20. Love and bless all your internal organs. Learn how to fall in love with them. According to the ancient healing Tao tradition, each organ stores different emotions. Your heart stores love and respect. Your lungs store humor, laughter, and courage. Your liver stores compassion and kindness. Your kidneys store gentleness and sensitivity. Your stomach, spleen, and pancreas store trust, faith, and hope. And your intestines store confidence.

21. If old thought patterns reappear, gently neutralize them as past history, no longer necessary. Evaporate these outdated feelings; see them disappear into nothingness. See them as old data that is now deleted from the computer of your consciousness. Use your breath to create space between these

thoughts. Imagine that as you breathe, your breath penetrates the area in your body where you feel these hurtful thoughts are located.

For example, if you feel some tension in your chest, imagine breathing into your chest, creating space, loosening the tension in that area and relaxing the muscles surrounding the tense area. Imagine rays of light penetrating the source of these patterns, transforming them to the light of love. Regain your joy—your birthright—and replace these old decisions. Avoid being restless or impatient as much as possible, because it is during moments of calm and peace that the forces of your new decisions work at their maximum. Practicing your new decisions daily with sincere motivation makes all the difference.

22.   Learn to listen to the signs your body gives you. When you feel slight tension, your body is telling you "no." You are allowing wrong thoughts to pass through you. Breathe and relax as you transmute, evaporate those thoughts to love. Gently shift your focus to your desirable thoughts, repeating them as your choice, shifting to feeling the sensations of your focused intention. You may wish to repeat the following:

"Let my decision to feel calm, quiet, joyful, loved, lovable, and loving move through me, my every thought, and my every action in every moment. Let it move! My trust in my new decision is strong. I rest my mind in confidence in my new choice. I know that it is good for me."

Or you may choose another decision that is more appropriate for your life at this time. Write it down, memorize it, or record it on a tape so you can listen to your own voice guiding you. It is valuable to listen to tapes, as you can let go more easily, without the need to think what to do next; let the tape guide you while the words do the work for you.

23.   After deep relaxation, repeat your new decisions over and over in your mind, imagining that you already live your life according to these new decisions. See how you move, how you feel, as vividly as possible. Envision what you say to others, what you wish them to say to you, how you live your life joyfully, with ease and kindness towards yourself. You may wish to

write down the script of your new life ahead of time so it becomes clearer while you do your practice.

I have included an Appendix of Healing Decisions at the end of the book to help you change your toxic attitudes to healing decisions.

Chapter 7

Step Four: Practicing the Daily Healing Routine

A colleague referred a New York physician with colon cancer to me one week before his surgery to have the tumor removed. I taught the physician an ancient self-healing exercise.

"But I don't reallly believe in this stuff," he pointed out..

"That's all right," I replied. "You don't have to believe in it. It still works as long as you do it."

Even though this advice seems to contradict my own beliefs, it's often been my experience that the faith the healer feels comes across to the patient and acts beneficially on him.

"But I'm going in for surgery next week," he continued.

"That's okay. Each time you do this exercise, imagine that when the surgeons open you up, the tumor is gone," I said.

"That's impossible!" he laughed, and then a moment later said, "It would be wonderful. I guess I have nothing to lose by doing it. I *will* do it!" A week later he called to announce that when the surgeons opened him up, the tumor was gone.

"Did you practice the exercise?" I asked him.

"Yes, I did," he responded.

"Did you practice the exercise five to 10 minutes, three times a day for a week?" I continued.

"Yes, I practiced it as you suggested," he assured me.

"Did you tell your surgeons about the exercise?" I asked.

"No," he said. "They were all surprised. I was surprised too," he added. "They called it a spontaneous remission."

This exercise is just one of the exercises in the Daily Healing Routine, which is the foundation of the *9 Steps to Reverse or Prevent Cancer and Other Diseases*. You can add or subtract any of the other exercises, but it is important to practice the Daily Healing Routine every day.

This is the healing routine that has worked for me and my clients and students. Eight years after the disappearance of my cancer, I still do a shortened version of this program because it makes me feel so good and healthy. This chapter contains a 20-minute version, a five-minute version, and a two-minute version.

The healing routine begins with deep relaxation.

The Benefits of Deep Relaxation

Feeling peaceful triggers the body's natural healing mechanisms, using its innate wisdom to heal itself. You will experience sensations of love and joy, which are the fuel that releases chemicals and hormones from the brain that strengthen the immune system.

Deep relaxation expands your heart's ability to give and receive love. When you open your heart, you find love within. Relaxation is the key that enables you to love people and your life, as well as yourself. You return to the awareness of your true essence—the love within your heart.

My first response to my challenge with cancer was, "I have done something wrong; I am being punished for something that I must correct." Learning to deepen my relaxation practice with each repetition opened my awareness to the understanding that sickness—including cancer—is just a message of love from my body. One of the things my body was telling me was to take time out to enjoy life and to take care of myself.

The benefit of regular deep relaxation is that it allows you to slow down and feel the enjoyment of the love that is in your heart. For some people it is easier to focus on God's love during relaxation. If this is easier for you, open your heart to receive God's love. Without the feeling of love, the heart shrivels and dies. To heal yourself, you need to open yourself to feel love. The deeper you let yourself go into the relaxation experience, the more love flows through you. *Relaxation opens the door to the love that heals you.*

At first, I, like many of my students, found it very difficult to take time to relax. There were always more important things to do. I thought, "I have to make this phone call; I must write this letter; I have to run this errand." The list of things I had to do was endless. I was last on the priority list, and the entire day went by without practicing relaxation. Only the threat of death forced me to drop everything and reverse my priorities.

In the morning as soon as I woke up, I did my relaxation practice. I remember making the decision to make work my last priority. "What good is all my work if my body is dead? If there is time left for work after I finish my practice, great; if not, too bad," I decided. The amazing thing that happened was after a few days of sticking to my relaxation and self-healing routine, I had so much energy that I did significantly more work more efficiently than usual, leaving more time for my errands, phone calls, and letters.

My clients use this exercise daily to prevent cancer or heart disease if there is a family history of these diseases. Clients have reported that doing this exercise three times a day not only improves their health, it calms their emotions. They tell me that they stop yelling at their children and their relationship with their spouse improves.

The following exercise is designed to help relax the body, mind, and emotions into a deeper level of trust and letting go to create the environment for healing.

Find a comfortable place to sit or lie down. Make this time of connecting with your body precious. Do not get up to answer the phone or to do anything else. Place a "Do not disturb sign" on your door if it will help. Imagine that you are in a place of timelessness. You have all the time in the world to be with yourself—nothing to handle, nothing to take care of, and nothing to think about.

Exercise: Relaxation Practice

To relax yourself, do the following four steps:

1. Begin by relaxing yourself as deeply and effortlessly as possible. Tense your whole body; feel the sensations of tension. Then relax; let go. Breathe in deeply and soothe any tension that is left using the breath. Notice the difference in your sensations. Note how it feels when you are more relaxed. Repeat this process as many times as necessary for you to feel

completely relaxed. Once you acquire the habit of doing it, your body will relax immediately, and you will only have to do it once.

2. Allow your breath to become quiet, slow, deep, and comfortable. Feel the sensations in your nostrils. As you breathe in, your nostrils feel a little dry and cool. As you exhale, they feel a little warm, soft, and moist. Allow your breath to become so quiet that you can hardly hear yourself breathing. Feel how smooth and even it becomes, with no pauses, gaps, or jerks in your breath.

3. Allow your eyelids to fall effortlessly over your eyeballs. Let your eyeballs remain motionless. Move to a neutral place where they do not have to do any work.

    Feel liquid love pouring from your heart as blood, feeding the cells with joy and nourishing them. The cells open and blossom, smiling at you with gratitude. Billions of your tiny little cells are filling their hearts and minds—the DNA and RNA codes—with your love. Joy, peace, and health penetrate the nucleus of each cell. Your cells radiate with health. Any diseased cell evaporates and a new healthy cell emerges. The cells are watered with the liquid love of the blood and the warmth of the sun shining love in the form of light from your heart.

    Seeds sprout and beautiful flowers emerge. Smell the fragrance, a divine scent you have never experienced before. Feel the pleasure and joy.

4. Bathe in these sensations. Allow your whole body to dissolve into this pure love. Stay in that melting state for as long as possible. Imagine that you are opening your heart to your beloved, using whatever image of your beloved that you see. Feel your beloved embracing you wholeheartedly, merging with your love. Celebrate this exquisite union. Allow your imagination to form images that make you feel deliriously happy.

    The energy of love is the most healing energy there is. It makes no difference whether your images are real or imagined; you can create that energy from within. Your beloved may be your higher self, someone you love dearly, your soul mate waiting to meet you, a saint, a flower, or whatever stimulates your feelings of love. Spend time exchanging energies with your beloved as often as you remember—a minute here and a few minutes there throughout the day.

Practicing this exercise for five to 10 minutes produces the best results. Five to 10 minutes of relaxation calms the body, and prepares you for the next three exercises in the daily routine. The length of time to relax the body varies from person to person. Start by doing the exercise for 10 minutes. With practice, you will be able to do it in five minutes.

Self-Healing Breath, or The Five-Minute Cure

This exercise has been a huge treasure in my life. I first learned it from a meditation teacher in New York in 1975, the year that my gynecologist told me that I had two fibroid tumors the size of eggs on my uterus.

"Can they disappear on their own?" I asked, wondering whether this exercise would make them go away.

"Only with the knife," he responded. "Without it, they will only grow bigger," he added. He made an appointment for me to come to see him again in six months.

"I will heal them with this exercise," I remember thinking to myself. I tried to focus and practice this technique, but could not do it. I'd either space-out, fall asleep, or forget it. A week before my appointment, I forced myself to concentrate fully to dissolve the tumors.

"Do it, please do it," I pleaded with myself. The thought of surgery frightened me so much that my fear enabled me to concentrate and do the exercise.

I dreaded going to the next appointment. When my doctor said, "The tumors are gone," I felt a surge of delight. I told him what I did, and I saw the words "she thought them away" written in his report. When I asked him for a copy of the report for my records, those words were missing. I asked him, "Why are the words 'she thought them away' missing? I saw you write them in your report." He did not respond. I was too meek and intimidated to ask him to give me a more accurate report. I let it go.

I felt very encouraged and thought, "Maybe it will also work on my allergies." I decided to give it a try. I had terrible allergies for 10 years and had to have biweekly injections in both arms. The injections helped somewhat, but I was still suffering tremendous discomfort—puffy eyes, runny nose, ceaseless sneezing, and difficulty breathing. Once I neglected to go for my injections, and I had to be rushed to the hospital. My face swelled up as though I was deformed. My ears became longer, my body was covered with a red rash and I could barely breathe. I was given an injection at the hospital that calmed me down. "Dare I risk having another attack if I stop the injections?" I wondered.

"How long do I need to continue taking these injections?" I asked my allergist. "For the rest of your life," he replied. The very thought made me feel depressed. A close friend of mine who was suffering from similar allergies told me that he had been taking these injections for 20 years and knew he must continue taking them for the rest of his life. That convinced me that there was no other way.

Nonetheless, I continued to practice the self-healing technique, and I soon noticed that my allergy symptoms subsided. I did not go for my injections, feeling an inner knowing that this technique was working.

Three weeks passed and I was fine—my allergies disappeared. "I did it!" I said as I jumped for joy. That was in 1976. I have not had an allergy attack since then. From time to time a small allergic reaction appears but as soon as I practice this self-healing exercise, it disappears.

I still practice this exercise when I go to bed at night and as soon as I awaken in the morning before I even get out of bed, because it is so powerful. It relaxes my body as I bathe in the beautiful energies this exercise produces, which keep me feeling blissful. I believe doing this exercise daily helps me maintain a youthful appearance. At 64, my hair is still dark.

Ever since I first learned this technique, I have been teaching it to others. The intention of the ancient healers who developed this process was to erase sickness and suffering from the planet.

In 1980, a nurse who faced arthritis and weight problems attended my workshop. After practicing this exercise for three weeks, Dina felt great relief. A year later, her arthritis disappeared, and she stopped taking her medication. "I also have been losing weight naturally without going on a diet. This exercise balances my body so I don't get as hungry as I used to."

"I have been teaching this self-healing exercise in the hospital to my patients and everywhere I go," Dina continued. "I find it to be the biggest help. A few years later, she told me that some of her patients with various diseases had used this exercise to heal themselves.

"What kind of diseases?" I asked.

"Asthma, back pain, high blood pressure, ulcers, all kinds of aches and pains, even colds and flu. I am now able to get rid of a cold in 10 to 20 minutes." Then she added, "I have also been able to teach this exercise to patients with heart disease and the results are impressive. They were able to clean out their coronary arteries and reverse their heart disease. Lifestyle changes, such as reducing stress along with this exercise have helped patients open their hearts to a deep level."

Last year, Dina called to tell me that her father passed away. "He was having a lot of pain so I taught him the self-healing exercise and his pain diminished. He passed away peacefully."

Over the years, I've changed the exercise to make it easier for my students and me to visualize. When I taught this exercise to Jack Canfield, the coacreator of the *Chicken Soup for the Soul* series, his response was: "I am filled with bliss. You should call it The Five-Minute Cure."

Exercise: Self-Healing Breath, or The Five-Minute Cure

Your solar plexus is a bundle of nerve endings. The word "solar" means "sun," and "plexus" means "center." Although Western medicine has not yet assigned a healing function to the solar plexus, ancient healers recognize this "sun center" as a powerful instrument in healing the body.

To use your breath for self-healing, do the following seven steps:

1. Breathe in silvery light, sunlight, or whatever image is easiest for you to visualize. If you can't visualize it, just saying the words usually works. Draw this energy—imagine it as liquid love—into your solar plexus, which is located beneath the diaphragm, above your waistline, and between the two halves of the ribcage.

   ◆ Take another breath, and as you inhale, draw this energy into the solar plexus as though it has nostrils that can breathe. As you exhale, direct this energy as though you were using your eyes to look inward and fill up the left foot, including the toenails. Breathe in the silvery energy, hold it for a second and fill up the left leg up to the knee. Breathe in and fill up the left thigh.

◆ When you hold the energy in the solar plexus for a second, you activate your nerve endings to transmit the energy like rays of the sun sending light in all directions.

2. Do the same with the right leg. The energy penetrates the cells as rays of love that heal, massage, rejuvenate, harmonize, and restore the cells to health. This energy is very healing.

3. Then fill your lower body, including the internal organs, your liver, kidneys, gall bladder, stomach, spleen, and pancreas. Then fill your upper body, including your heart and lungs. Fill the left arm, including the nails. Fill the right arm. Fill the neck and throat.

4. Breathe in the silvery healing energy through your solar plexus, hold it for a second and fill up the left side of your head, including the left brain. Now do the same thing with the right side of your head and the right brain. Then do the back of the head, the hind brain. Fill the front of your head, the forebrain and the face. Fill up your hair and aura like a halo surrounding your body. Now your whole body is filled with this energy, healing billions of cells.

5. Increase the energy you have been sending a hundredfold, like a tornado of energy, and direct it to the area you are healing—the area of the sick cells, cancer, or disease. You can send it anywhere to a physical illness, emotional pain, mental disorder, spiritual disharmony, or any source of stress you are experiencing.

6. The most important part of this exercise is *now*: In your mind's eye, see that area already healed and perfect, shining and vibrating with health, like a newborn baby, while you are sending extra doses of silvery light to that area. In other words, while

you are seeing the area as perfect, energize it with a beam of sunlight or silvery light flooding the area to give it the healing fuel it needs.

◆ New research in quantum science indicates that *we change what we see by looking at it.* Your inner eye emits a laser beam or radar that corrects the cells by merely seeing them as healthy.

7. Now, use all five senses. When you walk into the room of someone who has cancer, there is often the smell of decay. When someone is cured, there is the smell of freshness in the air. Imagine that you can smell that freshness in the affected area as if it has already healed. You may experience a fragrance that you have never smelled before. Taste it, imagine a delicious new flavor. Hear the sounds of peace and joy in that area. Feel the sensations. Touch them with your senses. The texture may be velvety or silky smooth. See the shape and the colors as if the area is healthy. Use all five senses while intensifying the doses of energy that you are sending to the area being healed.

◆ When you can begin to imagine in your mind that you are smelling and tasting the freshness of being healed and seeing, hearing, and feeling yourself as already healed, studies show that you are creating new synapses in the brain that then bring about your healing. Your brain responds to the images you hold in your mind. It does not care whether they are real or imagined. Chemicals and hormones are released *according to the thoughts and images we experience*, which are then registered in the hypothalamus gland, strengthening or weakening the immune system.

Do this exercise three times a day.

Healing Decisions

The third step in the Daily Healing Routine is identifying unhealthy decisions held in the subconscious that create cancer and other diseases and changing them to healing decisions. This step is essential to prevent disease from returning.

Because this exercise is for daily use, it is much shorter than the longer version featured in Chapter 6. If you wish to work more deeply with unhealthy attitudes, use the exercise in Chapter 6. Refer to the Appendix to help you identify toxic attitudes that have to do with cancer or other diseases and to see examples of how to change them into healing decisions.

Clients who practice this exercise report benefits ranging from reversing and preventing disease to enhancing creativity and improving their finances.

When I first saw a young businesswoman named Doris, she was overweight and her dominant hand was numb. "I was always made fun of in school since first grade. My mother would dress me in strange clothes, like a doll, and I wanted to hide. I felt terrible shame. I didn't realize that the decisions I made when I was a child were affecting my life today. I now understand the weight is my way of hiding this pain, so no one would know how I really feel."

Doris learned to make healing decisions that transformed her shame into self-worth. After practicing the Daily Routine, Doris lost substantial weight within a short time and the numbness in her hand disappeared.

John, a psychologist, attended a seminar to learn how to help his patients prevent and reverse mental illness, cancer, and heart disease. After using the exercises, John told me, "Identifying toxic decisions using your method has helped my patients clarify how they constantly beat themselves up. Identifying these attitudes seems to be half the battle. I have noticed a great shift in their awareness. Then it's easier to move them forward to tangible results.

"This exercise helps my patients meet the daily challenges they confront every day in their relationships and at work. One patient said that stressful situations no longer drained him. He stopped getting angry over little things and was able to listen to his children's needs more attentively. His creativity at work increased and his constant back pain of many years disappeared."

Changing toxic attitudes to healing decisions requires diligence and motivated practice. Your decisions need to be nurtured with daily love, like seeds planted in a garden. This way of thinking needs to be protected from self-doubt and negative responses from others, which can undermine your new, healthy perceptions. Just as weeds in a garden will overtake the flowers if not removed, doubts will crowd out healing decisions if not removed.

Practicing the next exercise for five minutes, three times a day will reinforce your healing decisions, protect them from doubt, and sustain them so they strengthen your immune system and your ability to heal.

Exercise for Healing Toxic Decisions

To heal your toxic decisions, do the following 15 steps:

1. Focus your attention on your emotions and the sensations you feel in your body as a result of cancer, other disease or emotional stress. Give voice to what you are feeling. If you are feeling anxious or fearful, imagine where you feel that emotion inside and the sensations associated with it, such as, "I feel my heart beating fast...butterflies in my stomach...tightness in my chest."

2. Ask yourself, "What is my attitude or the decision I have made that is making me feel this way?" Wait for a response.

3. Allow the feelings to spread throughout your body. If tears start up, give yourself permission to cry and feel whatever you feel as fully as you can.

4. Be open and vulnerable like a child. Tell yourself the truth. For example, "I am afraid that I will never get well and will never be successful."

5. Write down this attitude that your subconscious mind is holding on to. Identify as many of these decisions as you can.

6. Now choose healthy decisions as though this were the beginning of the rest of your life. How do you want your life to be from now on? Even if you think it would be impossible, remember that you can create your reality from this moment on *simply by envisioning and feeling the reality you wish to create.*

For example, you may choose to focus on the opposite of fear-based decisions, such as:

   ◆ Others have gotten well and so can I.

   ◆ The more I decide to believe that I deserve radiant health, the more it will show up in my body.

◆ I am getting stronger, healthier, happier, wiser, and more successful every day in every way.

◆ I deserve health, and others will benefit by my renewed strength.

7. Repeat your new healing decisions five to 10 times daily with seriousness and sincerity.

8. In your imagination, feel the sensations you would feel when you are in radiant health. Feel the joy and the love that flow through your body when you feel great.

9. Imagine that you are watching your life as though you were viewing a movie—with vivid images of yourself already being the way you wish to be.

10. Imagine what people say to you when they see you. For example, "You look so good. I am so happy to see you and to have you in my life."

11. Imagine what you will say to people when you are successful and in radiant health. Allow your heart to be your guide. Let it express whatever it wishes to express fully. For example, "I want you to know that I love you and really care about your well-being and happiness."

12. Imagine the expressions of joy, love, and caring on your face and the faces of others as they enjoy hearing you say these words.

13. Again, repeat your new healing decisions five to 10 times, *feeling* every word.

14. Fill the area where you felt sensations of fear with sensations of peace, joy, and love. Love that area. Love the fear. Fear was merely a message, feedback to let you know you had to change the decisions you made that did not serve you. *It was your body's way of reminding you that like everyone else, you deserve the best.* The sooner you know it and accept it, the sooner you will be able to reverse all the unhealthy decisions that have caused problems in your life.

Now, thank yourself for having the courage and determination to heal your life.

15. Repeat your new healing decisions five to 10 times three times throughout the day.

Connecting With the Wisdom Within

The wisdom in your body is amazing. Two cells—one from your mother and one from your father—combined into one cell and became you. All of the wisdom that was you was in that one tiny cell that was too small to see. This one cell split, again and again; split and split, and split, and split till it formed all your organs and your magnificent body. All the wisdom that you are is in every cell of your body. And *contained in each cell is the wisdom to heal.* Plus the body has the ability to heal itself.

When you cut yourself, how long does it take to heal? The body knows how to produce the right chemicals and hormones. Trust your body's wisdom to be able to heal itself. Learn how to get out of the way, to quiet your mind, to feel peaceful and joyful, and to fill yourself with the energy of love.

Develop your trust; cultivate your faith in the intuitive wisdom of your mind, body, and spirit. This knowing is born within you. All the wisdom or intuitive intelligence for healing your body is inside you. As you learn to connect with the wisdom within you, you learn how to receive guidance from your wise inner self to heal, increase your health, find solutions to challenges you are facing, achieve your goals, and create a better life. First, you need to exercise your intuitive muscles to develop your ability to listen and to practice taking action according to the messages you receive.

Following this intuitive wisdom is what allowed me to say no to any more surgery or chemotherapy and to begin the process of healing that restored me to radiant health.

In 1987, a beautiful fashion model named Helena came to me. She was suffering from hyperthyroidism, and her hair had started falling out. She was also having difficulty falling in love and forming a loving relationship with a partner. Every relationship ended in heartbreak and disappointment, either in herself or her lover.

"I sabotage anyone who loves me," she said as tears poured down her cheeks. "Either I attract someone that I feel is not good enough for me or someone who feels I am not good enough for him. I never win."

As Helena became more proficient in practicing the Daily Routine, her awareness grew rapidly. She reported, "As I was practicing the Wise-Self-Within Exercise, I received inner guidance that woke me up. I saw my fingers placed on my throat and heard the word, 'dishonesty.' I understood that my hyperthyroidism was a reflection of my not telling the truth. I realized that to survive as a child, I couldn't tell the truth. My father was violent and abusive, but we never talked about it. We pretended that it wasn't happening. And I still do it. It's a habit that's been very hard for me to overcome. Now I know this is the toxic attitude that has been causing all my problems and I can change it."

Helena developed new healing decisions. and, after practicing them, the hyperthyroidism reversed itself, and her hair stopped falling out. Her relationship problems also healed. She met a wonderful man. Helena is now happily married and has a beautiful teenage daughter.

Exercise to Connect With the Wise Self Within You

Practice this exercise after deep relaxation when your mind is quiet, your body relaxed.

To connect with the wise self within you, do the following four steps:

1. Sit or lie down comfortably. Breathe slowly, deeply, smoothly, and comfortably, allowing your body to relax. Melt into your chair each time you exhale.

2. When you are deeply relaxed, imagine that you can connect with the wise self within you. Accept whatever image shows itself to you. It may show up as a friend, a grandparent, a sage, God, a saint, a flower, a thought, a vibration, a sensation. There is no right or wrong way of doing this. Whatever image comes to mind is fine. Ask your image, "Show me what I need to know or do to heal."

3. Listen quietly for a response. If no answer comes, then open yourself more sincerely and ask again with a sense of seriousness. Ask for help from the universe, from a higher power, from God, or from your higher self. The answer may come later in a dream. Or you may hear someone say something and you will feel a sudden sense of "Aha! That is the answer for me."

The right answer usually comes with a feeling of knowing. All your senses give you signs. There may be goose bumps or heart palpitations or tears or a burst of energy. Pay attention to those signs. Our bodies speak to us constantly; we are just too busy to pay attention.

4.   When your guidance comes with an "Aha! This is the answer" experience, take action. Make a decision about when you will act according to the answer you received. And do it! That is when the magic appears. Synchronicity, new adventures, new people, and circumstances show up in your life and move you forward in your growth.

The more you practice this exercise and take action according to the answers you receive, the stronger the connection between you and the wise self within you grows. If you don't take action, the connection weakens, and you forget that you have the power within you to create the life you deserve.

I have recorded a tape of the Daily Healing Routine that I often listen to three times a day: morning, noon, and night. I find listening to the tape allows me to let go into deeper states of relaxation. This helps me focus more deeply on each word so it can easily penetrate the subconscious. I internally repeat each word I hear until I can feel it being absorbed into my cells.

Each morning before getting up, I lie in bed bathing in these beautiful energies, feeling each word to such depth that my body vibrates with delicious sensations. When I allow the words to move deeply within me, I feel as though I am hearing them for the first time. There is a new freshness and deeper understanding with each practice.

Practice the complete daily routine three times a day for 20 or 30 minutes, depending how much time you have.

A Five-Minute Daily Healing Routine

Once you are adept at practicing the complete Daily Healing Routine, I suggest you do a short version whenever you have five minutes. However, continue to practice the longer Daily Routine. This fast routine is not a replacement for the full routine, but you can also use it whenever you can spare five minutes.

Practice whenever you feel tired, anxious, or moody. Healing energy builds up and creates health. You will receive great benefit from devoting time to visualizing joy, health, and happiness in your life. My experience has shown me that *whatever we visualize clearly with feeling becomes our reality*. The clearer the image and the more you feel it, the faster the results. The more you practice it, the more it expands.

Many clients use the Five-Minute Daily Routine while undergoing chemotherapy to keep their hair from falling out, and others use the exercise for prevention, particularly if there is a history of cancer, heart disease or other serious illnesses in their family.

Exercise: Five-Minute Daily Healing Routine

To practice the Five-Minute Daily Healing Routine, do the following four steps, which includes relaxation, self-healing, affirming healing decisions and connecting with the wise, intuitive self, a minute and a quarter each:

1. **Relaxation:**

    Tense your whole body tightly, then breathe in deeply and relax. Do this three times. Let go and breathe in slowly, deeply, comfortably, and quietly. Feel your breath becoming quiet and smooth. Feel the sensations of the breath in your nostrils.

2. **Self-Healing Breath:**

    ◆ Breathe in silvery life-force energy, like bright light, from the universe into your solar plexus—just above your waistline between your rib cage and your navel.

    ◆ Breathe in, and hold the breath for a second. As you breathe out, direct the silvery energy down your left leg to the toes, filling your left leg.

    ◆ Breathe into your solar plexus, and hold the breath for a second. Then exhale all the energy down your right leg, all the way down to your toes, filling the right leg.

    ◆ Breathe in the silvery energy into your solar plexus. Hold it and direct it towards your lower torso as you breathe out, filling your lower torso with silvery light.

- Breathe into your solar plexus. Hold it, and direct the light energy toward your upper torso. Fill your entire upper torso up to your neck, as you breathe out.

- Breathe into the solar plexus, and direct the light energy down your left arm all the way to your fingertips, filling your left arm as you breathe out.

- Breathe into the solar plexus, and hold the energy. Breathe out down your right arm all the way to your fingertips, filling your right arm with light energy.

- Breathe into the solar plexus, and hold the energy. Breathe out filling your neck, face, back of your head and your whole brain with the light energy.

- Now breathe in the silvery light, and send it to the area of your body that is challenging cancer, sickness, or discomfort. See that area already healed—as perfect as when you were born—vibrating with health, surrounded by pure white energy or light.

3. **Healing Decisions:**

- Focus on the healing decision you are working on. Let your body be your guide to how you want it to feel inside. When something feels powerful to you, stay with it, and repeat it over and over inside in your own words. Here's an example: "I decide to choose to feel good inside, no matter what goes on outside of me. I can choose to feel calm, happy, and healthy."

- As you are repeating your healing decision, see yourself doing everything in life feeling joy in your heart, feeling calm, peaceful, happy, healthy, radiant, vibrant, and glowing with health. See it as vividly as you can as you repeat the words internally. For example: "It's good to feel good. It's fun to feel good. I love feeling good. I deserve it. It's okay to feel good."

- Be sure to complete this portion of the Daily Routine with these healing words or those of your choice: "My healthy cells know how to heal any sick cells. My body regains its natural state of health."

4. **Connecting With the Wise Intuitive Self**

The last part of the fast Daily Routine is connecting with the wise self within.

◆ Imagine that someone who cares for you very much is in front of you, smiling at you, giving you so much love. What-ever image comes to mind is fine. Focus on that wisdom, and ask whatever it is that you want to ask. For example: "What is the lesson of my disease? What is the blessing of this adversity in my life? Show me what I need to learn."

◆ Then listen quietly. The responses are there as soon as you ask the questions. We are not always ready to hear them; so sometimes it takes longer. Open your mind to receive the messages from the wise self. Pay attention to the signs your intuitive wisdom is giving you.

◆ When the answer comes with that gut-level knowing, it's important to take action. Make a conscious decision that you will use the answer you received to take action. Thank your wise self for this wisdom. Feeling the sensations of your body, gently open your eyes, feeling rejuvenated and better than before.

A Two-Minute Daily Routine

If time is really limited, you can also do the routine in two minutes— half a minute for each section:

◆ Half a minute of tensing the whole body and relaxing three times.

◆ Half a minute of doing the Self-Healing Breath Exercise throughout the whole body and seeing the area already healed.

◆ Half a minute of working on the healing decision by repeating and envisioning the new decision.

◆ Then half a minute of connecting with your wise self.

Practice for two minutes at a time when you are stuck in traffic, during commercials when you are watching television, or while you are cooking. When you practice two minutes throughout the day, each minute strengthens you and releases stress so that it does not accumulate. You release stress on a regular basis before it makes you tired and causes you pain.

If you don't have two minutes, try devoting one minute or 30 seconds to energizing yourself. For example, wear a watch that chimes every hour on the hour to remind you to practice the quick Daily Routine. Or you can place silver or golden stars where they will remind you to take a short energizing vacation. Your watch is a good place for a star. Every time you look at the time, you will be reminded to take a vacation from your busy life and do the quick healing routine. Or place a star on the refrigerator. Every time you open the door, you will remember. Also, the bathroom mirror where you brush your teeth, the mirror where you look at your clothes after you get dressed, your computer, and your desk at work are all excellent places for a star.

Exercise: A Two-Minute Daily Routine

To practice the two-minute daily routine, do the following four steps half a minute each:

1. **Relaxation:**

   Tense and relax your body three times; breathe deeply, slowly and comfortably. Feel love in your heart like the sun radiating light in all directions. Enjoy the sensations.

2. **Self-Healing Breath:**

   Breathe in silvery (or golden) light through your solar plexus; sending it to the left leg, the right leg, left arm, right arm, lower and upper torso, neck and head. Send extra dosages of energy to the area you are healing at the same time that you see that area already healed and perfect, shining and vibrating with health.

3. **Healing Decisions:**

   Repeat and visualize healing decisions, such as: "The more joyful I feel, the more my body heals. I choose to feel free to enjoy every second I breathe. I bathe in the energy of love of my breath that sends love in the form of oxygen to all the cells of my body. Any diseased cell is easily converted to a healthy cell."

4.   Connecting With Your Wise Self:

Breathe and relax into your inner knowing and ask, "Show me what I need to know or do to improve my health." Listen for a response and take action when you know you have received the answer.

Chapter 8

Step Five: Calling on the Doctor Within

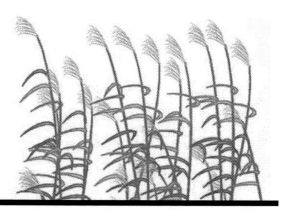

A neurologist, who is also the department head of a well-known New York hospital, came to me to deal with his fear of dying from disease. "So many people I know die from either cancer or heart disease," he said. "It's as if we have no choice, as though God unexpectedly points the finger at you and says, 'You'—and the next thing, you are dead. No one can predict who is going to be next."

He was also so traumatized by his fear of flying that he was unable to travel by plane. His wife was longing to fly with him to visit her parents.

I taught him the Daily Healing Routine and the Calling on the Doctor Within exercises. While practicing the exercises, he remembered an experience in his teens when he was traumatized by the death of a close relative. He also remembered that he nearly fell off a Ferris wheel.

He had an inner dialogue with the 15-year-old boy who was now able to verbalize this terror and identify the decisions that caused his fears. He made new healing decisions, which he practiced twice daily after deep relaxation.

I taught him the self-hypnosis exercise of counting backward from 50 to zero. "I saw myself on a screen in radiant health with a strong immune system that could easily identify and heal any sick cell," he said. "That made me feel very calm and peaceful. I then imagined myself flying with ease and comfort, free of anxiety or fear, enjoying my flight."

At the end of the fifth session, he felt good about his ability to prevent disease as well as the possibility of flying. A few weeks later, I received a thank you note reporting that for the first time in his life, he was able to fly. Feeling shaky at first, his confidence grew as he continued to practice the exercises. More than 20 years later, he not only flies great distances without fear, he no longer fears dying from cancer or heart disease.

The noted physician and humanitarian, Dr. Albert Schweitzer, said that within each one of us is a doctor who knows exactly what we need to do to get well. Step five is calling upon your inner physician and using its ability to heal your body. The exercises in this chapter allow you to work directly with the doctor within you to create healing. Plus, this doctor is *always* available for house calls.

Many of the exercises in this chapter utilize visualization to create internal changes. If you have difficulty visualizing, first practice the following exercise, which is intended to develop that skill.

Improving Your Ability to Visualize

Like many people, I found it almost impossible to picture images in my head when I first started doing visualization exercises. After practicing the following exercise, however, I now visualize easily, and my ability to see things clearly "in my mind's eye" continues to grow.

For those challenging cancer and other diseases, including mental and emotional pain, increasing your ability to visualize expands your ability to create a new framework so the changes in your body can take place. Research indicates that *when you visualize a change in the body, the body begins to adapt to that change.*

The Bible gives us an example of this in the story of Jacob. At that time, spotted sheep were the most valuable of all sheep. And because Jacob had very few, he placed spotted tree limbs where his sheep could easily see them as they grazed. When the sheep that were exposed to the spotted shapes gave birth, their babies had speckled fleece instead of the solid coloring of their parents.

The brain reacts strongly to the images we have inside our heads. It releases chemicals and hormones according to the images we see—even if they are just visualization. When we have calm, comforting images of feeling safe and protected, of experiencing pleasure, love, and joy, it releases chemicals that convey these messages to the rest of the body. When we have images of fear—of bad things happening, of worries—chemicals are released that place the body in the fight-or-flight response. The more the body is in that state of stress, the weaker the immune system becomes. *The more you focus on the images that make you feel joyful, the stronger the immune system becomes.*

My clients and students have had wonderful results using the following exercise. Some started out seeing nothing, but soon increased their visualization ability rapidly with practice.

Exercise to Improve Your Ability to Visualize

To improve your ability to visualize, do the following 20 steps:

1. Look around the room where you are sitting, and memorize what you see. Pay attention to the colors of the carpet, the floor, the ceiling, the furniture, and the other items in the room. Also pay attention to the clothes you are wearing.

2. Now close your eyes, and see if you can repeat the designs that you just saw—the colors, the shapes, the sizes of all you saw when your eyes were open.

3. Open your eyes and compare what you saw with closed eyes. Were you able to recreate those images accurately?

4. Again close your eyes. Can you now see everything you saw with open eyes with clearer, more vivid, accurate images? Do these first four steps several times before proceeding with the rest of the exercise. It is also helpful to practice them throughout the day.

5. Now imagine yourself in your favorite room. Close your eyes and imagine the furniture. Look at the ceiling. Look at the floor. What colors do you see, what shapes? Find an object. Take the object in your hand. Lift it up. Throw it in the air. Put it back.

6. Imagine yourself looking at your room from different angles, from different corners of the room. Imagine yourself up at the ceiling looking down at your room. What does it look like

now? Imagine yourself lying down on the floor looking up. What does your room look like from that angle?

7. Now, imagine that you are in your car. Imagine that you are holding the wheel. Can you see the dashboard? Can you see the windshield? See it as vividly as you can. Open your eyes.

8. Next, imagine that you are looking at a bright sun. What image appears to you? Is it a bright yellow color in a blue sky? Is it in the center of the sky or off to one side? Are there clouds in the sky? Imagine the shape, color, and size of the sun and of the clouds.

9. Now, imagine that you are on a beach by the ocean. Close your eyes and imagine the surroundings; look all around you. What colors do you see? Imagine the color of the water, the waves, the sand, the people, and the birds. Are there any trees? Imagine that you see a rainbow. Can you identify and see the colors vividly? Imagine its colors as sharply as you can—red, orange, yellow, green, blue, indigo, and violet.

10. Imagine yourself looking at the ocean at sunset or sunrise, at night and during the day. What images come to mind? Now, imagine that you see the moon. What image appears to you? Is it a full moon in the midst of clouds? Or a new moon in a dark sky?

11. Imagine your favorite fruit. Then imagine an apple, a pear, a banana, an orange, a grapefruit, a lemon, a grape, a mango, a papaya, a pineapple, a guava, and a strawberry. Imagine that you can feel the texture and smell the scent of each fruit. Now, imagine that you are holding and smelling a red rose, a yellow rose, and a white rose. Next, do the same thing with different colorful flowers of your choice.

12. Close your eyes. Feel the sensations in your heart while you imagine the shape of your heart and the red blood that is being pumped through it. Now bring the image of the bright sun into the center of your heart. Imagine your body turning into a blue sky and your heart becoming a bright sun radiating rays

of light throughout your body. Now, imagine a red rose in the center of your heart. Now, imagine your heart blossoming into a red rose.

13. With eyes closed, focus on the sensations in your body, and describe the images. What do you feel inside your stomach, in your chest, and in your head? Describe the sensations to yourself. If they are less than comfortable, examine the thought and belief behind the discomfort. Relax that area, breathe into it, and notice how the images change.

14. Close your eyes. Imagine that you are looking at your favorite pet. Touch your pet, savor the sensations you feel when you stroke it. Look at its eyes; what color are they? Notice as many details as you can. Now, imagine looking at and stroking a cat, a dog, a rabbit, a bird, and a fish.

15. With your eyes closed, imagine that you are eating your favorite food. Feel the sensations in your fingers as you hold your utensils. Imagine that you can feel the sensations of the food in your mouth. Imagine chewing the food in your mouth and savor the taste. Enjoy the sensations as if you are eating that food right now.

16. Imagine drinking your favorite drink and smelling its fragrance. Feel the sensations of pleasure as you swallow it. Now imagine drinking water. Then drink milk. Notice the difference in the texture and taste. Imagine drinking tea. Then drink wine. Notice the difference in the texture and taste.

17. Imagine drinking from different containers. First, drink from a glass, then a mug, a plastic cup, and finally a paper cup. Notice the difference in the sensations you experience as your lips touch each container.

18. Imagine a beloved family member sitting in front of or next to you. Imagine his or her facial expressions as vividly as you can. Imagine his or her smile, the clothes he or she is wearing, and the sensations you feel when you are with this person. Imagine hugging him or her. Feel the sensations of his or her touch.

19.   Now, visualize your mother. Can you see what she looks like? Imagine her in beautiful paintings, in the shades and colors of your choice. Create images of a nourishing, loving, divine mother nurturing you and feeding you with all you need. Bring that image of a loving, healing, divine mother into the area of your pain or sickness. Feel her love healing this area, stroking it with gestures of kindness, compassion, and real caring. Imagine that you are an innocent infant being held and rocked with so much love that you dissolve into that love. Imagine your body healed, your emotions joyful, your spirit enlivened, and your mind calm, wise, and empty.

20.   Practice this next step when you are with other people:

Look at the people around you. Look at what they are wearing. Close your eyes and recreate those images, shapes, and colors internally. Open your eyes and see if you remembered all you saw. Close your eyes again and see if you can remember what you saw more fully. Do you see the images any clearer now? Open your eyes.

Practice this last step as often as you can, whenever you are in a waiting room or in the checkout line. Know that your ability to visualize will improve with practice. For some people, it happens within a short period of time; for others, it may take longer. Even though I couldn't visualize at all when I started, after practice I was able to see faint images. I found that using my imagination to visualize made the difference—and helped me heal from cancer.

Self-Healing Disease

Research studies have indicated that the words we speak and the feelings they evoke affect our immune system. Using affirmations of health together with visualization can be very healing to anyone challenging cancer or other diseases. When you visualize with feeling, you manifest changes inside your body. Use whatever image works best for you. Some people like the image of a kitten roaming the bloodstream, hunting down and gobbling up the diseased cells. Other people prefer images such as a bolt of lightning blasting the tumor and healing the tissues around it. Experiment with different images until you find the ones that resonate with you the most.

This exercise has been very helpful for me as well as for my clients and students. I learned the first part of the exercise from Dr. Simonton and added a sentence from what I learned from Chi Gong master Dr. Zengo Yaul. I have also added images based on the feedback I have received from my students, images that helped them (as well as myself) feel that something was happening inside. When I was challenging cancer, I practiced this exercise daily. Now I focus on it every few weeks or months for maintenance.

Exercise: Visualization to Self-Heal Disease

To heal disease, visualize and repeat the following eight steps:

1. My white blood cells are strong, healthy, numerous, and a symbol of me. They are active and smart. They easily identify any diseased cell, and with a slight touch, they inject enzymes into the diseased cells.

2. The diseased cell walls collapse or return to a normal cell. The diseased cells are weak, confused, deformed cells that easily reverse their structure to normal cells with the love energy.

3. I focus on them. I can see them as a message of love, telling me to live my life more joyfully. I can see how the changes I have made in my life have served me well.

4. My white blood cells know how to heal the diseased cells. As an army of fairy gods and goddesses, they stroke the diseased cells with love, soothing them with a divine salve that helps them revert back to healthy cells. Or the cell walls disintegrate, and the debris is washed away by the urine and stools. New, healthy, radiant cells emerge in their place.

5. I imagine the tumor shrinking in size as I focus on it with the light of my inner eye. I imagine that ray of light acting as a laser beam directed at the tumor.

6. I watch it become very soft, and then chop it up into little pieces until it becomes liquid. I flush the liquid away with pure spring water. The liquid mixed with the water flows out the

pores of my skin and through my urine. The earth is receiving it with love as fertilizer.

7. The energy of love is filling the empty space where the tumor was located. Flowers in rainbow colors, representing the virtues of joy, wisdom, harmony, love, and peace, are growing in the area where the tumor was.

8. The area now looks healed and perfect, shining, and vibrating with health.

Helping Alleviate the Side Effects of Chemotherapy and Radiation

To help alleviate the side effects of chemotherapy and radiation, repeat and visualize the following seven statements:

1. The medical treatment is my friend, my ally, helping me heal any cancer cells.

2. My healthy cells are wise, very smart. They know to not allow in any chemicals. They know how to not absorb the chemicals.

3. They smile and gently direct the chemicals in the direction of the diseased cells.

4. The diseased cells absorb the chemicals and disintegrate.

5. The chemotherapy or radiation penetrates the sick cells only, eliminating these cells.

6. New healthy, happy cells are born in their place.

7. My body is getting stronger and healthier every day.

Self-Healing Tumors

This exercise is specifically for healing tumors—cancerous tumors, fibroid tumors, or any growth that you wish to eliminate from your body. Body, mind, emotions, and spirit are interrelated. If one part is out of balance, the whole system is affected. Pay attention to areas of your body that are crying for love. Send love, acknowledgment, appreciation, and healing to these areas throughout the day, every day, whenever you remember. Learn to listen to the messages they give you. If you have pain, I recommend practicing the pain exercise as well.

Exercise: Visualization to Shrink Tumors

To shrink your tumor, do the following five steps:

1. Imagine when you felt strong love for and/or from someone. Recreate that experience and feel those emotions right now. Feel the sensations of love in your heart. *This is the fuel that helps heal tumors as well as other symptoms.*

2. Imagine that you can breathe in and out through the tumor—as though each cell is porous and can breathe. As you inhale, the pores open up inhaling love in the form of oxygen into the heart of the cells. As you exhale, the pores squeeze out any debris, transmuting toxins to the divine elixir of love. Give the suggestion to this love energy to gently engulf the tumor.

3. Have a dialogue with the part of your body that contains the the tumor. For example, you may ask: "What is your message? What thoughts in my subconscious do I believe that you are reflecting?" Listen to your body's responses. Thoughts may appear in images of what makes you unhappy in life. Most people hold on to a belief that "if I had more _____ (fill in the blank, such as health, strength, friends, money, someone who loves me, etc.), I would be happy." That belief leads to frustration and unfairly causes you to be hard on yourself.

4. You may wish to make a new decision, such as, "I am willing to experiment with feeling happy whether more _____ (fill in the blank) shows up in my life or has yet to show up." For example, "Thank you for showing me that I am off balance in my thinking. I send you healing love vibrations for showing me the way. I accept myself as I am and am willing to be kind, gentle, and compassionate with myself more and more every day, every moment, with every breath. I wash my tumor with divine love from my heart. I accept a new reality of being a loving, nourishing being of divine

grace." You may wish to add anything that raises your happiness to higher vibrations of abundant health and aliveness.

5. Imagine rays of blue light, sharp as a laser beam dissolving the tumor away as it becomes liquid love. Feel this liquid eliminated and washed away through the urine and stools.

Keep on repeating this exercise three times a day, after deep relaxation in addition to the self-healing breath exercise.

Healing Disease Using Self-Hypnosis

The following exercise is useful in healing cancer and other diseases, and changing old thought patterns into healing ones. This exercise can be used to change the fear of disease into the joy of being disease-free.

Exercise: Self-Hypnosis for Healing Disease

To heal disease and change limiting ways of thinking with self-hypnosis, do the following four steps:

1. Close your eyes and go into a state of deep relaxation. Imagine a blank screen in front of you. Count backward from 50 to zero, moving deeper and deeper into relaxation, letting go more with each count.

2. When you reach zero, imagine yourself on the screen the way you wish to be: healthy, more radiant, more joyful, more tranquil, more energetic, more productive, more creative, more loving, more lovable, stronger.

3. Repeat your new healing decisions 20 to 30 times, sincerely feeling each word deep in the core of your being.

    For example: "I now know that I deserve to be successful in healing my body. I now own my power to feel good inside. Whatever goes on outside, I am in charge of my thoughts and my feelings. I choose to feel _____ (fill in the gap: calm, quiet, smiling, joyful, etc.)."

4.   To heal disease:

a. Repeat: "My white blood cells are active and numerous, an army of smart angels, fairy goddesses, or kittens (use whatever image appeals to you), roaming through my body and easily identifying any sick cell. With a slight touch, they inject enzymes into the sick cells. The sick cells' walls collapse or return to health. The debris is flushed through the body's systems, is filtered by the liver and kidneys, and then washed out through the urine and stools.

"My healthy cells are very intelligent, a symbol of me. My joy and enthusiasm is communicated instantly and directly to all cells of my body. I humbly ask my cells for forgiveness for treating them with less than the joy and respect they deserve. I forgive myself and ask for higher wisdom to help me accept it sincerely. The cells respond by owning their perfection, delightfully functioning in harmony, cooperating and collaborating with all the systems in my body. My immune system is enlivened and strengthened. My body's natural healing mechanism is activated and the wisdom that is within me guides me in the direction of wellness.

"My body knows how to restore itself. As I feel more joy, more love, more harmony, my body responds with more health and vitality. I look forward to full involvement with life. The more enthusiasm and passion I feel toward life, the happier my body feels and the faster the healing mechanism is triggered into action and dominance. I surrender to its wisdom. I honor, respect, and protect my healing decisions that help this healing activation. I love myself fully, absolutely. I feel secure, protected, comfortable, calm, full of pleasure. I feel reverence for these powerful energies. I nurture and nourish them daily, feeding them with my love, compassionately.

"My healing power grows and flourishes each time I practice this. Its potency multiplies abundantly. I am excited about increasing my well-being and feel thankful for the time and energy I invest in my well-being. My health is victorious. It is my natural birthright to be healthy, tranquil, and joyful. It is what life intended for me. I own my right to experience radiant well-being."

b. Ask the doctor within: "Show me what I need to know and do to get well."

c. Be still and listen to the responses within your body. The answers are always there, as soon as you ask the question. When the mind is calm and quiet, you will hear the messages. The problem is that our minds are so busy with outside events, thoughts, worries, and concerns that they cannot always hear the answers. Take time out to quiet your mind on a daily basis.

Relieving Pain

Cancer and many other diseases are often associated with pain. Having an exercise to alleviate the pain while you are healing is essential. People have been able to not only get rid of cancer pain, but headaches, migraines, back pain, emotional pain, and tightness in the body by using the pain-relief exercise that follows. Some people have been able to release their pain within a few minutes of doing this exercise. Other people need to practice it for longer periods of time.

Exercise for Pain Relief

To relieve your pain, do the following 12 steps:

1. Close your eyes; with your inner eye, look at the area of pain. Measure the pain from zero to 10. Zero means there is no pain, 10 means severe pain.

2. Now, feel the sensations in your eyes. Just imagine the sensations you feel in and around your eyes. Whatever comes to you is fine. There is no right or wrong way of doing it. *Just focusing your attention makes the difference.* Tighten the muscles of your eyes. Feel the sensations of tightness and then relax the muscles. Notice the sensations you feel when your eyes are relaxed.

Focus your attention in your face, head, and throat, and feel the sensations as you tighten those muscles. Tighten the muscles in your jaw, clench your teeth, and tighten your lips. Now relax them. Let the tightness go and feel the sensations of relaxation in your jaw, face, neck, and head.

Feel the sensations in your hands. Feel the sensations in your feet. Feel the sensations in your shoulders. Feel the sensations in your arms. Feel the sensations in your toes. Feel the sensations in your knees. Feel the sensations in your abdomen. Tighten your whole body. Feel the sensations of tightness. Now, relax your whole body. Feel the sensations of relaxation.

3. Feel the sensations at the center of your pain—be they physical, emotional, mental, spiritual—whatever pain or thoughts that are uncomfortable. Imagine that you can tighten your pain and the muscles associated with it. Focus your love on the pain and say, "It's okay, I love you." Vibrate the word "love" in the center of the pain. Imagine pouring liquid love that has soothing, medicinal qualities into the center of the pain. This healing liquid interacts with and absorbs the pain.

4. Feel the sensation of the muscles around the pain and allow them to relax. Feel the liquid love penetrating the area of pain. Allow the blood to flow in that area by opening it up; imagine that you can open that area. Breathe into the area of the pain. Relax the muscles inside and around the pain. Imagine space opening up in that area for energy to flow. Relax your veins and arteries. Imagine your blood becoming liquid love flowing in that region. Relax the center of the pain or the heart of the pain, where it hurts the most.

5. Have a dialogue with the pain: "What is your message? I really want to know. What are you protecting me from thinking? What are the thoughts that are so painful that the physical pain is preferable to those thoughts? I am now willing to face those thoughts."

6. Be still, and listen for the responses. By facing those thoughts, you can now use your wisdom to change them. You needed

the pain to protect you as a survival mechanism. It is now safe to know those thoughts. You now have the tools to heal them.

7. Feel the pain, exaggerate it, and allow it to spread. It may feel as though it is becoming worse. Don't be afraid to feel it as fully as you can. You are making it worse to really allow it to be felt. Imagine the pain melting into liquid then evaporating as steam becoming a ray of love as bright light. Allow the ray of love as bright light to spread throughout the room you are in, throughout the world, throughout the universe.

8. Release it into the universe as love. *You are changing the molecules just with your mind.* All you have to do is say, "Transmute the pain into love. Transform the pain into love. Change it into love vibrations. Evaporate it to a ray of love as bright light." See the molecules, electrons and neutrons all changing into the vibrations of rays of love and light. Envision it spreading throughout, releasing anything, any pain that's within, evaporating it, transforming it, and healing it. It becomes like beautiful stars, surrounding the whole universe.

9. Each time you exhale, squeeze out the air with the pain, evaporating it to love—as though your body is a transmuting machine that has the power to transform pain to pleasure and love.

10. Now bring back the rays of love to your body, into the center of the pain. Anchor the rays into a ball of bright light; your pain is now as bright as a sun radiating warmth and love in all directions. Imagine the light of the sun outside connecting with the light of the sun within you, feeding it with a constant flow of light.

11. Measure the pain from zero to ten. Zero means there is no pain, ten means very severe pain. Notice any changes from when you started the exercise?

12. Keep on doing this exercise: Open to the universe as you inhale, absorbing healing love energy into your body. Then exhale, squeezing out the air within you, transmuting, releasing,

evaporating toxins to love. Come back down deep into the center of the pain. Tense and contract your pain and your body, then relax. Open and expand, transmuting and releasing. Contracting, then opening, expanding, transmuting, and releasing. Opening, transmuting, releasing, and coming back. Usually, within five to 10 minutes there is a shift—the pain diminishes and often disappears. As you practice it, you will get better and better at it. Keep on expanding and contracting at your own pace.

Releasing Tiredness

All the chatter we have going on inside our heads is mostly nonsense, and it drains our energy. The loss of energy caused by this constant internal dialogue is what makes us feel tired. And when we are tired, it is easy to give up and not do the exercises that will bring back our health.

To release this wearying chatter, we need to first identify it. Learn to pay attention, to notice when this chatter starts inside your head. Be a silent witness. Don't judge or identify or cling to your thoughts. Don't give them energy by believing them. They merely show you what is going on in your subconscious, the thoughts that are blocking you from being healthy, free, radiant, and joyful. Don't force them away either. Gently let them pass by, like clouds that appear and disappear in your mind. Shift your focus to the sensations of calm in your breath. Maintaining a state of internal emptiness is best for recharging yourself. Being empty is very blissful, magical, and energizing.

Another way to quiet the chatter, release tiredness, and recharge is to try to predict what your mind is going to be thinking next. This allows the chatter to quiet.

Exercise to Release Tiredness

To release your tiredness, do the following nine steps:

1. Close your eyes and focus on your breathing. Connect the inhale breath to the exhale breath, and continue connecting the exhale to the inhale as though it's one long breath, with no gaps in between.

2. Now, focus on a color. For tiredness, I usually use the color orange. Use the color of your choice. Breathe in slowly and

comfortably, and as you exhale, let your whole body relax as though sinking into the floor. Become very still and quiet.

3. Imagine that you are breathing in sensations of being in love. That energy of love penetrates the molecules of tiredness—interacts chemically with them—transforming them into the divine nectar of love, as though you are inhaling the incense of love. *Aaaaah....*Good.

4. Now focus on your heart. Put your hands over your heart. Feel the vibration of your heart; feel it beat. Because the color red helps heal the heart, imagine red light, red fire, burning away tired or painful energy. Make the healing sound—*HA*—as you exhale to burn away any wounds, hurts, pain, heartaches, or harshness from your life. *Haaaaaaaaa.* Imagine them exiting out the top of your head, like smoke. *Haaaaaaaaa.* Use a higher tone. And again, one more time: *Haaaaaaaaa.* Good.

5. Now, look into your heart with a big flashlight. See if there's any darkness anywhere—any residue left of pain, suffering, discomfort, or anyone who's hurt you in the past. Using your imagination, invite that person into your room right now, and say out loud whatever you're feeling. Say it directly to them.

6. Exchange love from your hands to the heart and from the heart to the lungs, feeling the flow. Pay attention to this flow of love. This is your guide. These are your signs. If nothing is happening, increase the speed of your breath. Make the healing sound, *haaaaaaaaa, haaaaaaaaa, haaaaaaaaa,* and breathe from your mouth, speeding up the inhale and exhale. Every once in a while, about every tenth time, allow the *haaaaaaaaaaaaaaaaaaaaaaa* to be a lot longer, and let it out very slowly.

7. As you release any stuck energy in the heart, any tension, any stress, keep on asking, "What are you feeling, dear heart? What pain are you holding on to? What do you need?" Or whatever question comes to you. Either say it out loud or to yourself—whatever feels right. Keep the heart connection to the breath.

Breathe into the heart and release any heartache that is left from the past and again, say out loud anything else that comes to you.

8. When you release old feelings, it's important to fill that space with new feelings. Otherwise, there remains an empty space. Now, fill the heart with love, joy, compassion, and grace. Create an image of bliss, and surrender to that image of bliss. Fill your heart with that bliss, with good feelings, with ecstasy.

9. Talk to your heart, and express your gratitude to it for serving you so well for so many years. See it opening and blossoming like a beautiful flower. Imagine that you can smell the scent, the fragrance of the flower. Again, say the healing sound, *haaaaaa.* Say, "Bless you, heart; bless you. Thank you, thank you, thank you, heart. Bless you, heart. You're such a good heart." Once again, make the sound, *haaaaaa.* Imagine that your heart is opening. That it's blossoming like a rose. Touch the velvety texture. See if you can smell the scent of the rose in your heart.

Quieting the Mind

There is constant chatter in our minds. Whether we listen or not, the voices keep on telling their stories. These stories continue to drain us of valuable energy. They are meaningless and need to be quieted. You can deepen your ability to quiet the mind. Numerous research studies have proven the value of quieting the mind. When the mind is quiet, the body relaxes naturally and feelings of peace engulf us. *Feeling peace is one of the key elements necessary to stimulate our bodies to heal.*

It takes focused attention to quiet the mind. One way is to sit quietly, and listen to your thoughts. Another way, as mentioned before, is try to imagine what the next thought is going to be. See if you can predict it. You may notice you are able to keep your mind quiet for longer periods of time this way.

There are many methods for quieting the mind. A method that has helped me and my students is focusing on the words "my beloved," or on God's name—whatever name is in your heart—and repeating these words over and over internally with sincerity. Place your hands on your upper chest, near the heart, as you repeat these words. Some people find it helpful to connect with

God or a higher power that is close to their hearts. Other people find it helpful to focus on their inner child who has been wounded and needs love to feel good inside. Use whatever image works for you. With practice, the experience grows in meaningfulness, and the mind learns to be still.

When we are still, we are able to listen to the inner wisdom, to the doctor within, that knows what we need to do to improve our health. I have been practicing this exercise over and over thousands of times, and almost each time I do it, I feel moved to new feelings of delight and new depths of peace.

Exercise to Quiet the Mind

This daily exercise is best practiced on an empty stomach—before breakfast and before dinner—for 20 to 30 minutes, twice a day. The benefits are cumulative. Some studies indicate that one of the benefits of 20 minutes of being in deep stillness is that it is equivalent to eight hours of deep sleep.

To quiet your mind, do the following seven steps:

1. Create a quiet space where you will not be interrupted or distracted by phone calls. Put a "Do not disturb" sign on your door, or whatever works for you. Find a comfortable position to sit up or lie down.

2. Breathe in slowly, softly, deeply, and effortlessly. Place the palms of your hands on your chest over your heart. On each exhale, allow your body to relax, to sink into the chair or bed. Focus your attention on your nostrils. As you breathe in, it feels a little cold and dry; as you exhale, the breath feels a little warm and moist.

3. Locate a place inside your body where you feel perfect peace, perfect calm, like deep ocean water where there is no movement. Allow that calm sensation to spread all over your body, cell by cell, until you feel the peace dissolve into the stillness of your love.

4. When thoughts pass by, observe them as images on a movie screen. Then, convert them into the energy of love. Repeat internally, "My beloved, help me be only with you, clear these pictures from me. Love is how I know you, I want to know you." Do not identify or judge the thoughts as good or bad. Be a silent witness. "Aha, so this is what it is like to be a human being named [*your name*]; these are the thoughts that pass through

my head." Then come back to focusing on your breathing and your beloved, internally repeating "my beloved" gently, slowly.

Do not force the thoughts out. Allow them to flow out of your consciousness as you focus on your breathing and the sensations of well-being flowing through you. Thoughts stop us from feeling. When you focus your attention on breathing and feeling the sensations of love in your body, the distracting thoughts disappear.

5.   From time to time, focus on feelings of love for others. Remember the people in your life who you love, have loved, and have been in love with. Bring those people into the room using your imagination. Feel the intensity of love growing, feel the sharing, caring, and enjoying.

6.   Continue focusing on the pleasant sensations of your breath as you inhale and exhale. Notice how the breath becomes smooth and quiet, so much so that even you can hardly hear yourself breathing. Keep the flow of your breath even, with no pauses, no gaps, no bumps in the breath.

7.   Continue on your own for the rest of this practice period or until you wish to come back to full wakeful consciousness. Always leave a few minutes at the end of this exercise to do no work, to rest, to bathe in the sensations of pleasure. Observe the beneficial effects of this quiet time on your system, your body, mind, emotions, and spirit.

Activating Your Hypothalamic Orgasmic Response

Our bodies are miraculous. Everything we need is within the body. As I mentioned in Part I, a number of physicians, such as Deepak Chopra, say that all the medicines that we require are inside our bodies. We can manufacture everything we need. For example, by stimulating the hypothalamus, we can release hormones and chemicals that stimulate the pituitary gland to release its own hormones and chemicals, which then stimulate the adrenal glands to release their chemicals that strengthen the immune system.

In Psychology 101, we learned about the hypothalamus, which is a small area in the brain located in the center of the head. Studies were done where experimenters stimulated a certain portion of the hypothalamus in mice, and the mice experienced intense pleasure. Actually, they had orgasmic responses, and they loved it so much that they would rather have the stimulation than food. Some of them preferred the pleasure sensations to eating food until they starved themselves to death. One participant in my seminar said, "What a way to die; I'd rather die from feeling pleasure than from cancer."

While I was healing, I learned how to stimulate the hypothalamus by vibrating certain words while placing my focused attention in that area of the brain. Using imagery and the imagination, I would see beautiful words blossom as exquisite flowers. Suddenly I would feel chemicals being released and hear my whole body going, "Ah, this is beautiful." It felt really good.

Research indicates that the hypothalamus plays an important role in the health of the body. This gland can either suppress the immune system, creating disease, or strengthen it, creating health—*all depending on how we feel.*

Page 17 of The *Getting Well Audio Program Guidebook* states:

> "First, part of the hypothalamus—that part most responsive to human emotional stress—participates in controlling the immune system. Second, the hypothalamus plays a critical role in regulating the activity of the pituitary gland, which in turn regulates the remainder of the endocrine system with its vast range of hormonal control functions throughout the body.

> "...evidence suggests that the hypothalamus, responding to stress, triggers the pituitary gland in such a way that the hormonal balance of the body—mediated by the endocrine system—is changed. This is particularly significant since an imbalance in adrenal hormones has been shown to create a greater susceptibility to carcinogenic substances.

> "The result of such a hormonal imbalance can be an increased production of abnormal cells in the body and a weakened ability of the immune system to combat these cells."

As I mentioned in Chapter 1, research indicates that when feelings of emotional stress are replaced with feelings that give us pleasure, suppression of the immune system can be reversed.

The *Getting Well Audio Program Guidebook* goes on to explain on page 20:

"Once these feelings are recorded in the limbic system, messages are sent to the hypothalamus reflecting the altered emotional state....

"The hypothalamus in turn reverses the suppression of the immune system, so that the body's defenses once again mobilize against abnormal cells."

The hypothalamic orgasmic response is very healing because it releases medicines, chemicals, and feelings of well-being, which flow throughout the body strengthening the immune system. By letting go of our tensions and worries, we can relax and activate the pleasure response and feel bliss. Then the healing energy flows.

It's our thoughts and the feelings those thoughts evoke that influence our nervous and immune systems. You are free to choose whichever thoughts you believe are going to strengthen you. Thoughts that produce pleasurable sensations are good for us. *Harmony and gratitude, joy, and love are energies that liberate us from disease.*

You can choose to release the pain and the heavy baggage you've placed on your shoulders all these years that have made you feel bad inside. Feeling pain and suffering is like an addiction. It's erroneous learning from our past and from our society. Make feeling good a high priority, free of what others think about you.

We have been carrying others' problems on our shoulders, rather than putting our full focus on our feelings of well-being that will create improved health in the body. When we worry about others, we interfere with their journey. Our worry contributes to their negative perceptions of themseves, and we hold them back rather than allowing them to grow into their full potential. But when we see the magnificence in others—and ourselves—rather than the limitations, then we are free to blossom, each in our own way. Find ways to feel good inside.

As we feel and release this energy of feeling bad, it dissolves the energy jam, the blockage caused by emotions that have gotten stuck. You can melt or evaporate this burden, allowing it to dissipate into light. Allow yourself to be who you really are deep inside—full of goodness, love, and joy. Embracing and feeling this truth is the opening to pleasure and the path to health.

When I practice the hypothalamic orgasmic response exercise, I feel deep self-love. I don't need or want anything from the outside. I feel fulfilled and satisfied. Cosmic orgasmic energies start flowing through me that are quite exquisite and seem as though they release medicinal energies from within me. My body regains new aliveness. I experience a new expansion of health, awareness, and happiness. I jump with joy to do whatever task is at hand. I look youthful and glowing. When it happens, it feels as though this is the highest high I have ever experienced. Each time I reach a new high.

I discovered that orgasmic energy has amazing medicinal properties that help heal, rejuvenate, and recharge the body system. I have found that the energy of pleasure can help speed up the healing process. New electricity develops from the combined energies of pleasure and love.

Exercise: Activating Your Hypothalamic Orgasmic Response

To release the healing benefits of your hypothalamic orgasmic response, do the following 15 steps:

1. Close your eyes and breathe in the ancient vibration of love deeply into your heart. Breathe out the highest love to your body and the space surrounding your body. Do this three times.

2. Focus your attention on the hypothalamus, located in the center of your head. Feel the vibration of the word "pleasure" as you repeat it in the center of the hypothalamus several times. Then, feel the vibration of the word "blessings" as you repeat it in the center of the hypothalamus several times.

3. Imagine the hypothalamus drawing in bright light from the sun as you inhale. Imagine that the hypothalamus now becomes a small sun radiating light and love from its center. A halo of loving light shines brightly around it as it releases chemicals and hormones into the bloodstream and directly to the pituitary gland (located close to the hypothalamus) in the form of bright light, emitting sensations of pleasure. The pituitary gland receives this bright light with the message of pleasure and is transformed into a bright shining moon. The sun as the hypothalamus and the moon as the pituitary gland exchange pleasurable love vibrations as though joining in love with the beloved.

4. As you keep repeating the words "pleasure" and "blessings," feeling the vibrations of loving energy, observe how the sensations of pleasure grow within you. Empowered by the hypothalamus as a bright sun, the pituitary gland, the master gland that oversees the functions of the major systems of the body, releases its powerful chemicals. A bright halo of loving light radiates its message of pleasure and blessings to the blood and directly to the adrenal glands—which sit atop the kidneys in the small of the back—as the chemicals of pleasure and love pour forth.

5. Keep on repeating and experiencing the pleasurable energy of love as you repeat the words "pleasure" and "blessings" internally. The adrenal glands receive these chemicals of pleasure through the bright light, both from the bloodstream and from the direct connection with the pituitary gland. The adrenal glands become radiant moons with a halo of loving light surrounding them as an aura of pleasure. The kidneys receive this pleasure in the form of radiant light and blossom into brightly shining suns, forming a halo of pleasurable loving light around them. The adrenals release their potent chemicals that strengthen the immune system and calm your nervous system, allowing it to function harmoniously with the energies of the loving pleasurable light. The adrenals and the kidneys fall in love with each other and exchange love.

6. Continue repeating the words "pleasure" and "blessings" internally, vibrating that energy in the heart and lungs. All these bright lights of pleasure and love are transmitted to the heart as a new sun emerges in the heart and exchanges love with the lungs. The energies of love, pleasure, and blessings merge in the heart and the lungs as a bigger sun emerges from their combined energy exchange of love.

7. Imagine that your blood transforms into liquid pleasure and imagine love feeding the cells lovingly with the medicinal properties of the healing chemicals released. The billions of cells receive the messages of pleasure, love, and blessings as they transform their structure into radiant health throughout your body. The DNA and RNA codes become small moons

radiating pleasure and orgasmic love with the chromosomes, nucleus, protons, neutrons, and electrons of the cells that in turn are transformed into radiant moons and suns, joining in love with each other.

8. Imagine the organs and glands throughout the body lighting up with joy, falling in love with one another and making love. The tongue enlivens as the energies of pleasure, love, and blessings combine with the saliva to become an elixir of divine nectar emitted from the lovemaking of the tongue with the teeth and mouth. As you swallow this elixir of divine nectar, it becomes a healing ointment that lubricates and heals your body systems. Your eyes and ears liven up making love with each other.

9. As you keep repeating the words "pleasure" and "blessings" internally with sincerity, your brain brightens up and becomes the center of a huge sun making love with the internal organs of your body that have also transformed into many bright suns. Your whole body becomes a huge sun with a halo of bright, loving light surrounding it that is projected for miles around you.

10. Imagine the cells of your body, like billions of miniature *you*s, blossoming into beautiful flowers, smiling to you as they receive the warmth of your love generated from all parts of your body. As the cellular orgasmic response is triggered, all the cells regain their perfection. They return to radiant health and emit fragrances of joy, pleasure, love, harmony, happiness, peace, grace, humbleness, health, vitality, enthusiasm, passion, wisdom, and gratitude. The body is strengthened and empowered to be healthy, creative, productive, and to enjoy life fully.

11. Now, imagine eating pleasurable food. Enjoy each bite as though the food is making love to you and you are bathing in the vibrations of love and loving eating it.

12. Imagine the sky making love with the earth, and the earth vibrating with orgasmic smiles and growing delicious food with

which to feed you. Imagine the earth making love with the trees, and the sea caressing and making love with the sand.

13. Imagine that you are a walking soul, and the center of your chest is a moon, radiating gentle light that spreads for miles around you as a huge halo. Shift the light from gentle and soft to bright and intense to become a sun and then back again to become a moon. The moon spreads its light from the center of your chest; then the sun shines its light brightly. Imagine you are a dimmer switch turning on and off, dim and bright. Observe the pleasurable sensations your body emits.

14. Focus on the area you wish to heal. Stimulate and vibrate the pleasurable energies in that area. Surround that area with pure love. Visualize that area healing, releasing any stagnant energy that is now being evaporated to love. Envision that area regaining its natural perfection, radiating and shining with health.

15. Stay in the silence and simply observe the energies that are pouring through you in stillness. Remain in this state for several minutes.

As you walk through life, recreate these sensations of pleasure and love. Live for love; enjoy joining in love with nature and all there is. Walk in love. Ancient, ageless love is the most healing energy there is. Any time you feel negative vibrations or painful thought patterns, repeat the words, "All is love, all is blessed," to shift the energy back to the vibrations of love. Even if you don't feel it at first, it grows with practice. The more you solidify and maintain these sensations of pleasure and love, the more health is generated within you.

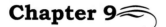

Chapter 9

Step Six: Using Your Doubt to Create Certainty

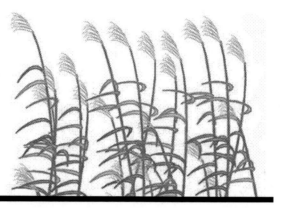

I once met the daughter-in-law of a royal princess who was suffering from lung cancer. When she heard my story of healing myself from cancer, she begged the princess to meet with me. At first she refused, not wanting to consider any alternative approach to medical treatment. Finally, she agreed to a short meeting. We spent an hour together, which rekindled her hope. "I would like to try your method," she said.

We worked together three hours a day for five days. Her husband and other family members also participated. We explored emotional responses to success and failure as well as thinking patterns inherited from her ancestors. For example, a subconscious toxic decision that had made it difficult for her to breathe fully and enjoy her good fortune was, "You have to be perfect; you must never embarrass us."

On our fourth day together, she told me how sad he felt that the dog she'd had for many years was dying. "We love him very much. He is like a member of our family," she said.

"What's wrong with him?" I asked.

"He has a large inoperable tumor on his head. I wish there was something we could do."

"Let's all hold hands together and do a healing on him," I suggested. We all held hands and I said, "We are now willing for this beloved pet to regain perfect health." They repeated the words after me. I instructed them, "Feel the sincerity of your willingness. Now allow your body and mind to become very still and quiet as you utter these next words. 'If it's in alignment for the highest good of everyone and everything, with only good consequences.'

"Now create certainty that this treasured family member is healed and perfect, shining and vibrating with health. Have no doubts; one tiny doubt can ruin the whole thing. Let's feel the gratitude that it is already done. And don't make a big deal out of it when you notice that he is fine. Be totally certain that it is done and give thanks."

The next day the dog was fine—the large tumor had disappeared.

A year later, I received a fax from the princess saying, "I am in good health." She went on to say that the most powerful exercise for her was Creating Certainty. "My family now creates certainty everywhere we go."

Doubt the Doubt

Step six uses your doubts about healing to create inner certainty that you *can* heal. Fear and doubt are the most prevalent emotions in challenging cancer and other diseases. Placing doubt in the doubts in order to create certainty has proven very helpful for me as well as my students. "Don't you think that there is a tiny grain of a possibility that the doctors misdiagnosed you?" I would ask. As soon as a student was able to say, "There is that chance, but very unlikely," I encouraged them to create certainty by visualizing the cancer gone, the tumor disappeared, the water in the lungs dried up, or whatever challenge they were facing gone. "Ignore the diagnosis," I would encourage them and myself. "Create a new reality, visualize it the way you wish it to be and create certainty. *It's the feeling of certainty that creates that outcome in the body.*"

During my darkest hours with cancer, doubts ran rampant. As soon as someone's face showed that "cancer is death" expression, my doubts that I could heal myself were triggered. When doubts and fear took hold of me, my symptoms became worse, and that in turn created more fear and doubt. It became a vicious cycle. When I stopped the live-food diet and wheat grass juicing program, my fear of having to stay on it for the rest of my life was greater than the fear that if I stopped the diet, I would die. Both fears weakened me.

Then I thought I was doing great. My pain had diminished, my lymph nodes were normal, and my tumor had shrunk. "I'm on the right track," I assured myself. I was feeling elated, playful, and enjoying my life. "Cancer was sure a blessing," I thought. "It taught me how to let go and feel good inside about myself and my life.

Then out of nowhere, I remembered my doctor's words, "Yes, it is cancer. You must go to the hospital right away, or it will soon end your life." Or I would recall the remark of a well-meaning relative, "You have a nerve not to do chemotherapy. Who do you think you are?" Or I would remember a mocking remark, "She thinks she can heal herself."

Waves of fear would start passing through me as strong as electric current—and all my doubts reappeared. I would tell myself, "You are fooling yourself. You must have surgery, radiation, and chemotherapy. This is not a joke, you must follow the doctor's recommendation." An image passed through my mind of my friend who died of breast cancer after she had surgery and chemotherapy. More thoughts and memories of doubt surfaced.

Before I knew it, I started feeling strange symptoms once more. "That's it, my cancer is back, or it never really left me. I deluded myself." I would start feeling so bad that quite rapidly my body would deteriorate—as though it was decaying in front of my eyes. I almost believed that there was nothing I could do to reverse it. "I tried everything, and nothing really works," I decided.

Many old, unhealthy attitudes would reappear, such as a pattern of finding things to blame myself for. "I didn't smile at this person," "I should finish that," "I should have known better," and so on. Somehow, I thought others' problems were my fault. An old conflict with a friend who was challenged by heart disease passed through my mind. "I shouldn't have had that thought. Maybe I was jealous, and that's why her health is failing." And on and on.

My situation got worse. Feeling desperate, hopeless, and helpless, I remembered my wise inner self. "Show me what I need to know and do," I asked my wise self.

It told me, "Practice what you teach, doubt the doubt."

I noticed that as I focused on those words, my body started relaxing. I understood the message my body was giving me. "That's the sign from the wise self." My heart leapt with joy, feeling hopeful once more.

My wise self continued, "Don't believe everything you hear. You don't have to do anything if it doesn't feel good."

"What a relief." I breathed a deep sigh. "I can choose to believe what makes me feel good, loving, and joyful."

I then challenged each of my doubts and inserted doubt into each and every doubt. Next, I imagined the white blood cells—numerous healthy wise cells that easily identify any sick cell—and with a light touch, injected enzymes into the sick cells. The sick cells' walls collapsed and healthy, new, radiant, and smart cells were born instead. I knew that this was physiologically accurate, and it helped me imagine myself to be a big, healthy cell injecting enzymes of doubt into the sick, harmful thought patterns of doubt. I felt the doubt disappearing and my energy of joy returning.

I focused on inserting doubt into the doubt and creating certainty by affirming these statements:

"I doubt that cancer has returned. I choose to believe that I can heal myself. Others have done it and so can I. I choose to remember how good I felt. All I need to do is take time to rest and do my healing work, and I will feel great again. I am daring, independent, self-reliant, and courageous and prefer to be this way rather than be dependent on others' thoughts, opinions, or beliefs to show me the way.

"I can doubt what the doctor told me I must do. I tried surgery and chemotherapy, and it is clear to me that it is not my path. I enjoy being on my path more than following others' paths, even if they are medically trained. Medicine is good up to a point, but it does not address the whole person. It is still in a process of evolution, and eventually physicians will study or need certification in psychoneuroimmunology. Some physicians are already doing just that.

"I doubt that my friend died because it was too late for treatment. My friend in all probability died because she was miserable. She hated her life, and she wanted to check out. She was too embarrassed to talk about her pain. She had no one to turn to. Had I known then what I know now, I could have helped her. I forgive myself for not knowing.

"I doubt that it is my fault that whatever goes wrong in other people's lives has anything to do with me. Other people have their lessons to learn and their own journeys through life. It is not up to me to save them. They can save themselves. I know that the happier and freer I feel, the more energy I have to heal. Then I can be an inspiration for others to do the same.

"I doubt that I tried everything. There is huge wisdom within me. Try tapping more deeply into that source of help, and watch what happens.

"I doubt that I will not be respected for my belief that I and my higher power can heal myself. It's my life. I can choose to respect myself no matter what feels right for me to believe in, whether others approve of it or not. What they think and believe is their business, not mine.

"I doubt anything that makes me feel uncertain about myself. The more I cultivate confidence and trust my inner knowing, the more certain is my ability to feel good. The more I feel good, the faster I can heal myself."

Within a short period—sometimes just a few hours, other times a few days—I would regain my certainty. My vital energy emerged and I was back on my way to recovery. In November, 1995, my doctor confirmed that the cancer was gone.

Creating Certainty

The doubts you have about yourself are in direct proportion to your ability to create certainty about healing yourself. What you choose to believe in and create certainty in is your choice. So the work is to go deeply within and see where you still doubt yourself. For example, "I'm not good enough. I will be made fun of and ridiculed if I walk around with certainty that I can heal myself. Someone will be jealous, envious, or uncomfortable seeing me filled with certainty and may then find ways to hurt me or put me down."

Typical doubts that pass through the mind are, "Who do you think you are? What makes you think you are so great? Shame on you! You are nothing." Or you may remember overhearing someone saying, "She thinks she knows how to heal herself, but she doesn't." Even if you have heard others make these comments about other people, these statements enter your consciousness and insert the sensation of doubt into your mind.

Think of all the people in your life who might have given you such messages intentionally or inadvertently. When you feel doubt, feel the pain in your body, a slight tension in your shoulders, in your stomach, or in your heart. Feel the fear that is hidden underneath the feelings of doubt. You may notice that your body tightens up when you dwell on doubting yourself. The tightness may be quite subtle and unnoticed because it is deeply ingrained in your subconscious. It is important to allow these feelings to emerge as fully as possible. If you deny them or brush them aside without working them through, they will continue to fester inside you. Breathe deeply into those sensations and observe the thoughts that pass through you as you do that.

For example, "If others see me as confident, they might fear losing control and may have to challenge me. They may feel threatened by my new wisdom. They won't like it. They may become mean and use anger to intimidate me. They may blame me and make me feel miserable." Feel each thought that passes through, the tightness and pressure each image produces. "If I express what I feel and think, I will be rejected and then I will reject myself, and that will hurt the most."

Have a dialogue in your mind with those images or thoughts. Such as, "Why would you do that to yourself? Why would you reject yourself?" Then wait for a response. A response may be: "To please others, so they will like me and not reject me. If I doubt myself, they will see me as weak and will not bother attacking me." And so on. Go deeply within these areas of your subconscious.

Breathing deeply and slowly into the areas of tension helps reveal these unconscious thought patterns. You may remember incidents in your childhood when you were rejected when you expressed yourself. Perhaps you were shamed by a teacher in school or made to feel small and humiliated by others who did not know what they were doing.

Have an inner dialogue with those people who have treated you this way. Imagine one of them sitting right in front of you. Look that person in the eyes, and tell her how that situation made you feel. For example, "When you said that to me, I felt like there was something wrong with me. I twisted inside and my body felt tight, defending against attack. I felt as though I just had a knife go through me. It caused me to suffer over how inadequate I might really be." Then ask her, "Was it your intention to make me feel bad about myself?"

Then imagine changing seats; you now become the other person. Feel what it feels like to be the one who said those words that caused pain, and then respond as the other person. You may say something like, "No, it was not my intention to make you feel bad. I was just trying to get your attention."

Now switch seats, and be yourself again. Don't judge or hold back anything. Allow your anger to rise up if you wish, allow your hurt to be exposed, and cry if that feels right to do. Imagine speaking to the other person until she understands how her behavior made you feel. You may say something such as, "When you speak to me that way or in that tone of voice, it makes me doubt myself." Or you may choose to feel your anger more fully, and with a strong tone of voice, say, "Don't you dare speak to me like that! I deserve better than that, and I insist on being treated with respect." It may feel awkward at first to say whatever you feel like saying, even knowing that you are not going to be punished for your courage.

Now imagine switching seats again and become the other person. Feel what it feels like to hear the words that were just said. You may respond with something like, "I'm sorry if I said something that hurt you. I wasn't trying to make you doubt yourself. Please forgive me. That was never my intention." Switch seats again and be yourself.

To insert doubt in the doubt, it is helpful to continue with the dialogue until you feel a resolution, a feeling of comfort. After you have experienced fully and have said everything that came up for you to say, you may have a healing dialogue. You may say something like, "I want to feel love for you and for myself. When you say things that make me feel hurt, I stop feeling my love for myself. And I don't feel good about who I am. Then I stop feeling my love for you, and I don't feel good about who you are. I forget all the good things that I do like about you and all the things that I like about myself." Or anything that will make you both feel whole and allow the sensations of love to flow. You might say something like, "If you weren't trying to hurt me, what was your good intention?"

Imagine switching seats again and being the other person. You might say, "I was totally focused on what I needed to do and was just trying to get it done. I never intended to hurt you. I'm so sorry. My intention is just to love you."

Then switch seats again and allow yourself to receive this communication. Take a moment and breathe it in. Allow yourself to let go and release the hurt and pain. Forgive the other person and then yourself.

It is important to start the internal management. If as a child you received a big dosage of criticism that made you feel unhappy, then every little thing can trigger that pain to resurface and you'll begin feeling those old doubts. As your self-doubt is triggered, you will also doubt your new healing decisions.

It is helpful to delve deep within your consciousness and remember the very first time you learned to feel doubt about yourself. What images come to mind? Look inside and ask yourself, "How much do I doubt myself, and how does it show up in my daily life?"

Soon you'll be able to say, "This is what I was feeling and experiencing at that time, and this is what I feel right now." Write it down. Then challenge each of these statements. See what evidence you have to support those statements. Challenge the insecurities that the doubts created.

Self-doubt is a result of the accumulated messages from your past that you took into your heart and believed. Whether it was to please others or because you had no choice as a child to think differently, it can still affect you now—until it is worked through and healed. As you create certainty about who you are and about your right to feel joy and love, your self-confidence and health will grow.

Melinda, a housewife who was challenged by cancer, told me how she remembered a little girl in nursery school calling her names: "You are dirty. You are an asshole," and how when she heard those words, she burst out crying. As she was growing up, she always felt there was something wrong with her. She remembered being constantly criticized by her teachers, parents, and siblings. She learned to internalize her feelings of shame and self-blame.

She was convinced that she was hopelessly to blame for everything that went wrong in everybody's life around her. She became shy and withdrawn, continuing the pattern of self-blame without knowing it. She married a man who treated her the same way she was treated in childhood. She was so used to being blamed for others' frustrations and disappointments that she did not question it. She kept on blaming herself subconsciously. She felt a lot of emotional pain for many years until she was diagnosed with breast cancer.

While practicing the exercises, she was able to reverse the self-image she had developed of herself based on early childhood incidents. As her self-image improved, she started smiling and laughing more often. Even though she did go through surgery, she feels good about her life and is certain that cancer will not reappear. She understood that cancer was giving her a message of love, telling her to change the faulty self-image she had to one that reflects who she *really* is.

Changing unhealthy decisions to healthy decisions, as well as creating certainty exercises, is best done when your energy is high. When your energy is low, take it as a sign to relax and ask the universe for help. That is a good time to do just your relaxation practice with no extra exercises.

I started to pay attention to when my energy was high and when it was diminished. I learned to stay away from toxic people with their fears that brought me down. I moved towards people who loved me, and I felt love for them. I noticed that watching certain programs on television made me nauseous and fearful, while other programs were uplifting and made me laugh. The one program I always watched and felt uplifted by was Oprah Winfrey's show. There were many times I found myself wasting my good energy and not being aware that I was doing this until I felt weak and exhausted. I learned by trial and error. When my energy was high, I was able to perform amazingly well in all levels of my life.

Exercise to Insert Doubt Into Your Doubt and Create Certainty

To create certainty by putting doubt in your doubt, do the following eight steps:

1. First, identify the belief or attitude you are holding in your consciousness that makes you doubt yourself and your ability to heal. For example, if you are challenging cancer, you may have the attitude, "This cancer will kill me, and nothing can help it heal." One way to identify your attitude is to focus on whatever pain you are feeling. For example, fear and doubt are a form of pain just as all negative emotions are a form of pain. To begin to heal that pain, exaggerate it, wallow in it, make it worse, let it spread throughout your body, be with it, cry it out. Crying is very healing; it melts blocked energy. When you cry, the belief or attitude will emerge.

2. As soon as you identify the attitude, write it down and watch if any additional thoughts show up. For instance, "I will die a horrible, painful, torturous death." Keep on identifying what other painful thoughts you believe in. Write them down.

3. Now one at a time, put doubt into those thoughts; challenge them with new healing thoughts, and practice believing these new attitudes. For example:

    ◆ Others have healed from cancer, and so can I.

    ◆ The thoughts I choose to believe in make a significant difference.

    ◆ I can choose to feel calm and quiet; I can smile on the inside.

◆ I am in charge of my thoughts and my feelings.

◆ Many doctors have made mistakes. There is a tiny grain of possibility that the diagnosis was wrong. I am open to the possibility that I am disease-free.

◆ Many people have been diagnosed with "spontaneous remission" when their doctors discovered their disease was gone. I choose to be one of these people.

4. The way to create certainty is to repeat these sentences or your own— over and over with sincerity—using the phrase, "I am willing." For example, "I am willing to allow _____ into my life" (fill in the blank) or "I am willing to open to the possibility that _____ ," (where you might fill in, "I am deserving of feeling good inside and regaining perfect health.").

5. In your stillness, feel the truthfulness and sincerity of your willingness—no movement. Be with this willingness totally, be one with it. In your mind's eye, see yourself and feel the sensations of when the doctors tell you, "A miracle has happened— your disease is gone!" I remember visualizing and feeling the emotion of joy when I imagined my doctor saying these same words to me. When it happened, I was so certain and used to feeling that feeling from practicing it daily, that it did not feel like something new. Certainty creates "a matter of fact" kind of knowing—it does not need to be proven. It is best not to make a big deal of it.

6. Protect your new attitudes until they become as strong as trees. Water and nurture them daily with much love, repeating and visualizing your affirmations with joy. Imagine them to be beautiful flowers planted in your consciousness, in the space between your atoms and molecules. Imagine a variety of flowers emitting fragrances that you enjoy, growing to become huge, powerful fruit trees. It is better not to tell people about your new beliefs; their doubts are contagious. When you are strong, you can then share the fruit of your tree with everyone.

The path to health is feeling more joy, more peace, more harmony, and more love. This is the emotional fuel that triggers the body's systems to function in balance and harmony. You can choose to experience these sensations as often as you wish. It is your choice.

7. If doubts show up, write them down. Challenge them by placing doubt in them. If you have to trick your mind to create certainty, do it.

8. Be creative in your own way to *feel* certainty with all your senses. Smell it, taste it, see it, feel it, be it, hear it, touch it, know it, own it—without a shadow of doubt. Do it with ease and grace, effortlessly, as a matter of fact. *When you hold that reality to be as real as any other reality, it gets manifested. It's your choice to choose the reality you wish to have in your life.* I remember often saying to myself, "Even if it's not true, it feels so good to believe it that I don't care. I have nothing to lose by believing it, probably everything to gain." And choosing to believe in a new reality gave me back my health.

Practice your new affirmations of putting doubt in your doubts three times a day. For best results, do this after deep relaxation. Some studies suggest that the new attitudes of certainty penetrate the subconscious mind after 21 days of regular motivated practice. Some research indicates that it takes about six to eight weeks to change attitudes with sincere practice. I recommend 10 to 20 minutes for each practice, three times a day.

Chapter 10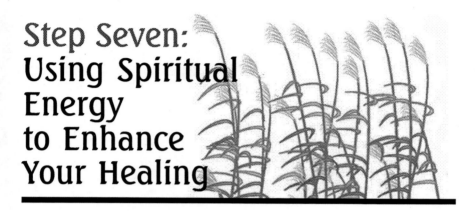

Step Seven: Using Spiritual Energy to Enhance Your Healing

For most of her life, Karina suffered severe back pain, and she was also distressed about having writer's block. "I want my creativity to open up," said this 40-something mother. "Writing is important to me, and I don't know why I am so blocked."

Then she confided the sexual fantasies she needed to reach orgasm. "I can only have an orgasm if I have fantasies of being abused by a man. I am so ashamed of myself, and I wish I didn't need to use such fantasies," she said, shaking with embarrassment.

I suggested she practice the exercises in this chapter. "The wise self within you will show you how to heal the blocks in your life."

She breathed a sigh of relief.

Using these exercises helped her explore the source of her need to imagine being abused to feel turned on sexually. While practicing the exercise to connect to a higher source, Karina had a breakthrough. She remembered an incident in which her wealthy father forced their cleaning woman to have sex with him. Karina was only 4 years old, but she remembered feeling sexually turned on and having an orgasm as she heard the woman from the bathroom pleading, "No, please don't, sir. Please don't."

"I sobbed helplessly when I suddenly remembered that day," Karina admitted to me. "It was as though my brain opened up, and for the first time, I understood. Now it all makes sense. The first sexual experience I had—where I felt sensations of sexual pleasure—was associated with abuse and fear. Since then, part of me has been blocked by images that haven't permitted me to honor and respect myself.

"I opened your book to see what exercise would help me heal this issue. My hands felt like they were being divinely guided to the exercise on using the power of focused intention. I began practicing it daily. Within a few weeks of working on forgiving my father for his cruelty and releasing those images, my back pain diminished rapidly—and I was able to reach an orgasm without having to use abuse fantasies."

A few years, later Karina reported, "I released the writer's block—I've just published my book!"

Step seven is reconnecting with your goodness and the most powerful source of all healing—your spiritual core or pure love. Know that the highest part of your being is goodness, beauty, truth, and pure love. Remember, the feeling of love triggers the immune response and releases the chemicals and hormones that produce healing. The exercises included in this chapter are designed to facilitate accessing and using this most valuable healing resource.

Accessing the Love That Heals You

Because the healing energy of love is of paramount importance in reversing and preventing disease, it is vital that we learn to tap into this precious commodity. The place to begin is by loving ourselves.

I often hear my clients say, "I believe that I need others to love me first so that I can then love myself. How do I change that belief?" This is a common misconception. We often feel that the love we need to feel better about ourselves and to accelerate the healing process has to come from outside ourselves. That is not the case. The truth is that we all have access to the love that can heal because it resides *within* us. And we have an unlimited supply when we learn how to access it.

It is helpful to remember that your source of love does not depend on someone else. Others can love you only to the extent that they love themselves. The more they love themselves, the more they are able to feel love for you. On the other hand, the more they hate themselves, feel guilty, angry, and irritated, the more they hate you, blame you, are angry with you, and get irritated with you. *It has nothing to do with you; it is their journey.* They need to learn to love themselves just as you need to learn to love yourself. You may wish to practice the healing attitude, "I am willing to open to the possibility that I am lovable and that it is safe to feel love for myself."

The reason to love yourself is not to please others so they will love you. The truth is that the less you love yourself, the less others will love you. *You love yourself so that YOU are filled with feelings of love and joy, which then creates healing in your body.*

Often, people feel embarrassed by feelings of love and try to shut them down. Thoughts such as, "Will I be taken advantage of or rejected?" block the flow of this valuable healing resource. A healing attitude to counteract that toxic thought is, "I trust the wisdom within me to know how to act firm when needed, while benefiting by feeling the flow of deep love fully within me. The more loved and loving I feel, the more loved and loving I become."

"What if I love and don't feel loved back?" I often hear my clients say. This is another toxic block to accessing the healing energy of love. The antidote to that toxic thought may be, "The more I experience the sensation of love, no matter how others respond, the healthier and stronger I get."

We sometimes blame ourselves when we don't feel loved. A client told me, "When I thought that my love was not returned, I felt pain. Then, I held my love back for fear of giving what was not wanted. I started doubting myself. Maybe I'm not loving or lovable." Those doubts caused a constriction in the center of her heart, which later showed up as heart disease. She shut down her heart to avoid feeling the pain of rejection. However, the pain of denying self-love caused a greater pain.

Underneath our doubts, there is usually a toxic attitude that there is something inherently wrong with us. This destructive attitude disconnects us from the love of our true self. Accessing the love within allows us to reclaim our self-esteem and to be lovingly healed.

Nicole, a stunning model living in New York, wanted to overcome her fear of staying home alone when her husband was traveling. She felt such severe panic that she was incapacitated with terror. She had a friend stay with her while she was working on healing her fears.

Her best healing occurred when she devoted time to spiritual growth. While practicing the spiritual exercises on a daily basis, Nicole not only healed her fears of staying home alone, she fulfilled her deepest longings.

"I live in this beautiful penthouse, yet it is not important to me," said Nicole. "I am the happiest when I feel unattached to everything, with no desires whatsoever, except the presence of the Divine. I could live in a cave and enjoy my life just the same when I feel connected to my true self. Then I lose interest in trying to get what I want. The truth is, the reason I wanted things from the outside was so that I could feel this joy. When I feel connected to my inner essence, I feel that joy. I don't have to struggle to get things from outside of me. I feel the most confident in myself when I let go of who I think I should be and just merge with my true self."

She added, "There are days when I lose that contact, and I start looking for someone else or for some material thing to make me feel good. The more I practice the exercises, the more I love doing them because they bring me back to myself, and that's the place where I enjoy being the most."

"When I focus my attention on that Divine presence within, I feel most connected to my inner joy" she commented. "What was most helpful for me was feeling unattached, resting in the light and love of my soul, and allowing my higher self to run my life for me. Insights that helped me understand my fears would appear spontaneously.

"For example, I noticed how I form my opinion about myself according to what others think of me rather than what I think of myself. When I allowed other people's thoughts to affect me, I would feel miserable, and the fears would appear. The more I feel connected to the goodness of my higher true self, the more I realize that what I think of myself is what really counts."

Exercise to Access the Love That Heals You

To access the love that heals you, do the following four steps:

1. Repeat these healing affirmations three times a day:

   "I accept and love myself just as I am. I approve of myself free of conditions that constrict the flow of my love. The more I sincerely love and respect myself, the more love flows joyfully throughout my body. I deserve to feel my love. I know that it's good for me. I feel better than ever before when I allow my love to flow in my heart, my blood, my bones, my cells and every part of my body where disease has been. I love myself. My highest, true self is pure love. I am willing to open to that knowing and feel it. I am love. I am love. I am love."

2. Feel the love in your heart. Feel this love flowing throughout your body, filling you with healing energy.

3. Send love to your wise, true self within and feel it coming back to you. You are feeling the love of your highest, true self.

4. See if you can experience the presence of your true self inside you. Feel the love that you are.

    When you focus on the love in your heart, it expands and flows throughout your body. The purer, more genuine, and intense the love vibrations you feel, the more the energy of love helps heal your body.

You will find that as you focus on this love in your heart, you will access the wellspring of love deep at the center of your being (it has sometimes been called spiritual energy) to enhance your healing.

Connecting to a Higher Source

Connecting with my spirit, my spiritual true self, or higher power has helped me heal the most. Many blessings appeared in my life. One of the blessings was a new sense of courage to open my mouth and ask for what I wanted. I have always been very shy, but suddenly I found myself speaking up.

For example, while I was working as a staff psychologist in a mental health clinic, my supervisor, who had trained me in Gestalt therapy, told me that he'd been invited to London to teach Gestalt therapy to a group of professionals.

"May I come teach with you?" I heard myself blurt out the words.

"You are welcome to come if you can pay your own way," he responded with a grin.

Teaching with him opened new doors, which moved my life in wonderful new directions.

9 Steps for Reversing or Preventing Cancer and Other Diseases

In 1993, when I was experiencing the most intense terror of death from cancer, changing my old decisions about death to a spiritual understanding learned from my wise inner self helped me heal those panic attacks. My body would jump at night in terror, feeling nausea, and my heart would race with the thoughts that I was going to experience a terrible death. As soon as I identified the beliefs I was holding on to, my panic stopped.

"Aha, so that is what you believe," I thought, smiling to myself. "You don't have to believe it if you don't want to. You can choose new decisions that make you feel calm and joyful." I worked on the new decisions three times a day, and my fear of death disappeared.

I had become extremely successful as a psychologist. In spite of that, there was no understanding or support for the magical, spiritual journey I was experiencing. Mostly, I was met with ridicule and sarcasm from family, friends, and colleagues. Gradually I started doubting my own experiences, and the spiritual life that filled my soul with joy diminished until cancer woke me up in August of 1992.

I now know that it was a wake-up call, a message of love from my soul, urging me to realign my life with my true self, my passion, my purpose, my mission. Because of my cancer, I became more fully aware of my mission. Each time I would talk about the possibility of erasing sickness, pain, and suffering from humanity, my eyes would start overflowing with tears of joy. It felt as though sparks of energy would burst out the top of my head like fireworks. I knew this was a sign from the wisdom within that I was on the right track.

Pay attention to these signs. They show you the directions that will enhance your life. Taking action according to these signs is extremely important.

On a daily basis I connected with the wisdom within and asked, "Show me what I need to know and do next." For example, I would have a thought, "Go for a walk on the beach." I took action and went for a walk. I was amazed when I found a pile of stones that were carved like letters spelling out words. The words spelled, "You love all." So that's what I need to do next, I thought to myself. I knew I needed to practice increasing my feelings of love toward "all." That was my work. The benefits of taking action based on this spiritual guidance were fulfilling and moved me back into alignment with my higher self.

Exercise to Connect With a Higher Source

To connect with a higher source, complete the following six steps:

1. Sit comfortably or lie down. Breathe in a soft, warm, loving, and relaxing breath. Exhale deep love, and share it with your spiritual source or higher self.

2. To access a higher spiritual source or your higher self, it helps to imagine an enlightened, spiritual teacher or master or your God in front of you. You may think of Jesus, Mary, Moses, Mohammed, Buddha, Krishna, Elijah, or any other saint, sage, or a friend you trust that you know really cares about you.

    One way of knowing whether the image is the right one for you is the sensation you feel or the energy you experience when you think of that person. When you feel sensations of peace and calm, you know that you have chosen the right image for you. You can also imagine your higher self in whatever way it shows up for you.

3. Imagine yourself merging with the energy of love of that spiritual teacher.

4. Imagine telling that teacher all that is in your heart. Expose your pain and be as honest as possible, as though you are talking to a therapist or a healer sitting right in front of you. Express any fear, anger, resentment, or frustration in your life.

    We often walk around feeling angry with people who have upset us. We can get caught up in anger, revenge, or annoyance.

5. Whenever these thoughts show up, direct them to your spiritual teacher or your higher self instead of the people you are upset with. Simply shift the focus from their image to your teacher and say how upset you are as if he or she is that person. Let your teacher be the one who absorbs the negative energy and transmutes it to love. Tell the teacher about your fears, your worries, your desires, your aspirations, and fill your body with the energy of love of your teacher.

6. Surrender to that love. Allow yourself to dissolve into the spiritual vibrations emanating from this Divine love. Take as much time as you need until you feel recharged.

You can practice this throughout the day, whenever upset feelings or thoughts interfere with your feelings of joy. If someone has hurt you, trust that the universe is just and that person will learn the lesson h or she needs to learn. You don't have to drain your valuable energy by focusing on dialogues that stir you up inside.

Using Spiritual Energy to Heal

Spiritual energy is a lot wiser than you might think. There is help available to us that cannot be explained with the rational mind. But the heart knows. Listen to the voice of your heart, to the love that is deep within your heart. Your heart has the wisdom to guide you on how to heal your body and your life. Be here now in this moment. This moment you can open your deep heart to feel this love. When the door is open, walk through. Feel the love in your heart even if you think your actions are not perfect. Know that most of the wisdom comes to us through our mistakes—bringing greater understanding, compassion, mercy, peace, joy, love, and support. Be just as you are—fallible, vulnerable, and open. The more you open your heart, the more fully the healing energy flows.

Exercise to Use Spiritual Energy for Healing

To use spiritual energy for your healing, do the following four steps:

The word "God" in the following exercise refers to a higher power, infinite intelligence, the universe, or pure love. Use whatever name resonates with you.

1. Repeat the following with reverence, seriousness and sincerity. You may use your own words; this is just a guideline.

    "In your name, my beloved God (or whatever name resonates with you), help me heal this divine body, this holy temple. Help me discharge the sickness, the energy that is negative. Help me to be Your hands, Your heart, Your eyes, voice, and love. Reveal to me who I am. Help me be an empty vessel because You are the knower, You are the healer. I align myself with the purity of the vibrations of the most high, allowing them to pass through me as an electric current that heals."

2. Place the palm of your right hand a few inches away from and facing the area you are healing with the left palm facing outward. Bring in healing energy from the universe, rotating your right palm in a circular motion to loosen up the stagnated energy. Imagine the energy of disease evaporating to love and being released out of your body to the universe through the left palm.

3. Use the sound *haaaaaaaaaa* to help convert the energy to love.

4. Imagine the healing energy passing through the area to be healed as a color. Use whatever color appears in your imagination. Each color has a different value. Some studies indicate that the color green helps heal the muscles and bones; blue heals the soft tissues, such as internal organs (liver, kidneys, heart, lungs, etc.); and yellow gives you energy. However, whatever color feels right to you will give you the benefits you need.

According to Dolores Krieger who developed the Therapeutic Touch Method based on research studies at New York University, using color energy had healing effects on mice, plants, and humans.

Moving the Life-Force Energy in Your Body

The ability to move the life force energy in your body with your inner focus is valuable for many reasons. Painful emotions cause the muscles to contract. This constriction then makes the blood flow inharmoniously, thus blocking the energy flow. When the blood flow is constricted, the energy gets stagnated and does not move freely. The exercise that follows helps you learn to connect with the energy flow within, releasing blockages that were caused by emotional pain. This energy flow within the lower spine is known in the yoga traditions as the kundalini or life force. As this energy moves up the spine, health and spiritual abilities grow. For example, it becomes easier to maintain a healthy, flexible, youthful body, while other abilities manifest, such as intuitive guidance.

This exercise has helped my spiritual growth and my ability to move the energy within me more freely.

Exercise to Move the
Life-Force Energy in Your Body

To move the life-force energy in your body, do the following eight steps:

1. Sit up straight. Ask a higher power or your spiritual guide for help.

2. Imagine yourself in sound health, living life with more passion, excitement, and enthusiasm.

3. Feel these energies opening in your heart, blending with the love that is there. Open your heart and your love to absorb these energies fully.

4. Using your breath, direct the energy of love—as if it were wet and moist and with a rainbow of healing colors—up your spine, slowly, softly, with kindness, gentleness, compassion, feeling moved inside, with tears of joy pouring out from the colors.

5. Let the muscles relax in your legs, your arms, your abdomen, chest, face, throat, and scalp. Let your mind relax.

6. Direct the energies to move up to the top of your head and form a fountain about 12 inches or more above your head, showering the space around the body, your aura, your spiritual body with these colors of love.

7. Smell the fragrances, touch them, see them, and taste them. Hear the sounds of love and joy all around you. Continue doing this until your body is filled with images and the energy of bliss.

8. Melt and dissolve into this blissful space until your body feels peaceful, calm, tranquil, and serene—so much so that it feels as though your body has disappeared.

Using the Power
of Focused Intention

I learned in India that there is an unseen power to the sound vibrations of certain words considered sacred. For centuries throughout the world, people from every spiritual tradition have felt connected to a higher power when sacred words were spoken. The repetition of these potent words only makes them stronger.

If you feel comfortable, repeat your sacred words during deep relaxation and repeat your new healing decisions; both can help anchor the new beliefs faster. It is a cohesive force that fills in the space that is created by releasing old patterns. The vibrations of these sounds solidify new, healthy patterns in the subconscious. It's a form of focused intention or prayer.

Research has shown the power of prayer. In his two ground-breaking books, *Healing Words: The Power of Prayer and the Practice of Medicine* and *Prayer Is Good Medicine: How to Reap the Healing Benefits of Prayer*, Dr. Larry Dossey demonstrated that prayer heals—even at a distance. He did a double-blind study that showed how prayer and sending energy can actually heal people who do not even know about it. The people who were praying knew nothing about the people they were praying for except their name and their age. The results of the study showed that there was a significant difference in health improvement in the people who were prayed for, while the other people in the study stayed the same or got worse.

One way to use focused intention is to go into deep relaxation and repeat the words of your choice, while adding your new healing decision. This cohesive force helps anchor a new belief on the cellular level. Use the words that you feel comfortable with. Repeat God's name or whatever name is in your heart. If you feel that God does not exist, I recommend a deeply spiritual phrase or word such as *pure love, peace* or whatever fills you with the highest vibrations. Repeat it constantly or as often as you remember. However, 24 hours a day is best. Tell your brain to repeat it while you're sleeping, talking, or working. In difficult times, it will protect you.

Saying a prayer of focused intention is a way of anchoring faith and trust in your body. Repeating sacred words was like magic to me; they helped me have faith that I could heal from cancer. To this day, the more I cultivate faith and trust within me, the more my life blossoms. Many sacred scriptures say that God is love and love is God. A master teacher from India, Babaji, has said, "Pure love is so powerful. It is the anti-atom bomb." Opening the heart to pure love or God's love heals the soul, which is the most beneficial healing of all. Can you imagine a love so intense that you feel you are in love with the most perfect lover? That love is the fuel that makes our hearts sing. *Love is the fuel that not only makes our bodies release chemicals and hormones that give*

us a pleasant feeling of calm and a euphoric high, the release of these chemicals also strengthens the immune system. Intense love is magnetic energy that not only heals, it attracts and magnetizes your heart's desires to you.

Do not let a day go by without praying to your spiritual source and asking for your heart's desire—your full, radiant health. Then repeat the name of God ceaselessly and feel the love restore your health.

Here is an example of an exercise in focused intention—or create your own prayer, one that has meaning for you.

Focused Intention Exercise

Speak these words to your spiritual source with sacred reverence:

"Dear beloved God (higher self, life-force energy, or all there is), Show me how to be one with You. I want to love purely, unconditionally, totally, and freely, to love as You love. Please show me how to do that, and give me the wisdom and the strength to follow through.

"I ask to be free of negative emotions of all kind—free of anger, jealousy, guilt, shame, blame, misunderstanding, unhealthy competition, upset, or conflicts. Show me how to stop comparing myself and my life with others. Show me how to be pleased with my life, knowing that all is in divine order.

"I know that when I feel bad inside, it is old patterns of self-hatred. I know that these negative emotions are merely indicators telling me that I am resisting wellness, resisting feeling Your love, feeling joy, celebrating life and allowing my desire for radiant health to materialize. I know that as I relax and allow Your life-force energy to flow through me, radiant health is my natural state of being and my aspirations are manifested.

"Help me heal these patterns within me and become an example to others that it is possible to be in radiant health and in total love. Help me see others' wholeness and perfection, let me be free of judgments or of feeling superior or inferior.

"Help me see the spirit within me and within everyone I meet rather than being stuck in their imperfections, weaknesses or old personality patterns. Help me be a pure vessel of your light, of your love, of your joy. Help me to be empty of thoughts that drain my energy, and instead fill me with the energy of bliss that is my birthright.

"Fill me with the energy of pure, radiant health. I ask for Your blessing to pour down upon me now. Thank You, beloved God. Thank You for blessing my life."

Chapter 11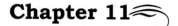

Step Eight: Following Your Heart's Bliss and Living With Passion

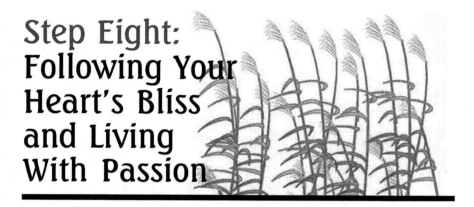

Sam had been suffering from bouts of depression while challenging heart disease, and he was finding it difficult to function. His breathing became extremely heavy each time he climbed a few steps. He felt that he was living his life without purpose, and, furthermore, he hated his job as an accountant.

While practicing the exercise for Creating Bliss and Finding Your Passion, he was surprised to feel joy. "I had a clear image of spending time in nature, working with horses and feeling very happy and fulfilled. I had no idea my heart's longing was to be with horses in nature."

A few weeks later, Sam and his wife drove to a horse ranch near their home to check it out. It seemed like the same location of where he'd seen himself being in nature while doing the exercise. It mirrored his experience so closely that he decided to accept a part-time position working there. Over the next few weeks, as he spent time caring for the horses he loved and teaching people how to ride, his depression disappeared.

A few months later, Sam's wife told me, "He's found his passion and has been a delight to live with since he started his new job." Sam added, "No wonder I was depressed all the time. I was forcing myself to do something full-time that I hated. I discovered that I can do both. I've opened a private practice as an accountant, choosing my own hours to work part-time, which I like because I am balancing it with what I love to do." He found this combination of jobs satisfying and joyful. As he followed his heart and his passion, his life became worth living again. Two months later, his angiogram showed that there was no longer anything wrong with his heart.

Following Your Heart's True Bliss

When you follow your heart's true bliss, you reconnect with your true self—your goodness, love, value, and joy. These are the feelings that strengthen the immune system, which bring you back to health. When you follow the longing of your heart, you will feel bliss that will enliven you. You will feel loving kindness and incredible joy.

These sensations of joy release chemicals and hormones from the brain strengthening the immune system. The hypothalamus gland registers the sensation of joy and releases chemicals that send messages of peace, calm, love, safety, protection, comfort, and harmony. As these chemicals flow throughout the blood, all systems of the body function harmoniously. The blood pressure is perfectly regulated; the digestive system works efficiently, the breathing is slow, smooth; and calm; and the body manifests health.

On a daily basis, I choose to follow the longing of my heart. Every day, I ask my heart rather than my mind to be my guide. For example, when I wake up in the morning I automatically practice the self-healing exercise while still in bed. This energizes me with feelings of joy. I go for a brisk walk for half an hour or more. This helps my cardiovascular system get active. I then ask my heart, "What would you like to do next?" I then follow its guidance.

Usually the guidance is to have fun with whatever work I need to complete that day. To have fun with the things I find challenging, such as paperwork, I imagine that I am watching a movie being entertained by this person called me. Then, the paperwork becomes an easy task.

Next, I reward myself by breaking for lunch. I eat slowly, fully enjoying the taste. I chew each morsel of food at least 50 times, as I have learned from the macrobiotic method of healing. I read a book about a man who healed himself from cancer by chewing each mouthful of food 200 times.

Following my bliss sometimes takes me on unusual adventures. I try to make as few plans as possible ahead of time to leave room for spontaneous events to occur. For example, when I was visiting Los Angeles, I was planning to celebrate the New Year 2000 in Colorado. Then my friend told me that he was going to Maui. My heart lit up when I heard the word "Maui." "How wonderful," I thought. "I wish I could go." But I dismissed it because I'd already made plans to go to Colorado.

As I was waking up on the day I was scheduled to fly to Colorado, the word "Maui" passed through my mind. My heart opened, and I felt such sweet energy of soft love that it woke me up. "Follow your bliss," I heard myself say. I jumped out of bed and changed my flight. Wonderful synchronicities and magic happened during the two weeks I stayed in Maui. The magic of those two weeks has continued to this day—I eventually moved to Maui and made it my home.

At first, it was very difficult for me to follow my heart's bliss. I would feel guilty just thinking of doing that. What helped me the most was to ask myself daily, "If I had only a few weeks or a few months to live, what would I do? How would I spend these days?"

I decided to stop worrying about finances, cut down on my work and expenses, and live a simpler life. Giving up my financial security was very frightening at first. I bought a home in India for $5,000, and then an inexpensive motor home in Colorado. It calmed my mind to know there were less expensive ways to survive than what I was used to. I also discovered that yoga centers, ashrams, or healing centers, which are located all over the world, were other options for alternative living. There, you can live free in return for a few hours of work each day. Tao Garden in Thailand is one example of a beautiful and inexpensive healing center.

The primary goal is that you live within your means and not spend more than your budget allows.

Soon, my priorities shifted and it became easier to follow my bliss. I decided to spend more time with my family and friends that I loved. I started traveling more often to Israel, where I was born, to fulfill my soul's yearning to spend time in my native land. I spent a lot of time with my son, celebrating his being in my life. Each day I would ask myself, "What will bring me joy today?" I let my heart guide me.

I remember visiting many doctors for routine checkups. One day I asked myself, "Is this what I want to do with my time—waiting in doctors' offices—or would doing something else give me more joy?" I remember responding, "It would give me more joy to swim with the dolphins and watch movies." I got up and left the office. I came to Hawaii and now swim with the dolphins whenever I feel pulled to do that. I have not needed to visit doctors for many years.

Become very in tune with your body. If you feel a little off course, take time out and increase your self-healing routine. I regain my health quite fast when I do that. I find spending time in nature, going for walks on the beach, hiking in the mountains, and connecting with the spirit of nature to be blissful. I regularly keep in telephone contact with my family and friends all over the world. I spend time with supportive friends who are nurturing and loving. All of this is what makes my heart fill with bliss.

In 1996, I asked my wise self to guide me to what would be blissful for me to do next. I got an immediate response, "Fall in love with someone."

"That *would* be fun," I admitted to myself. But the next thought that passed through my head was, "You have only one breast. Remember, no one is going to fall in love with you with one breast."

"Aha!" my wise self responded. "So that's what you believe, do you? Well, change that belief."

I changed that belief by choosing a new healing decision that I am not my breast, and I deserve the most wonderful man in the world. Within a few days of practicing this new decision, I met a wonderful man. We fell in love, and we had a spiritual wedding with dolphins and whales. We stayed together for six months.

Then we realized that our paths were very different. I forgot about my own life's work to erase sickness and suffering. I got too involved with his life. He was the one to see it first and said, "I am blocking your progress, and I don't want to take that responsibility."

I was amazed to discover that it did not take me long to heal my broken heart. Doing the exercises in this book helped me transfer the intense love I felt for him to feeling intense love for my inner self. The six months we spent together felt like 100 years of love, a whole lifetime's worth.

It was time to move on, to fulfill my mission, and write this book. Had I stayed with him, this book would never have been written. Now, I am open to being that intensely in love with every human being. That is my true bliss—to be in love with everything and everyone.

Living With Passion

Finding our passion for life or our deeper life's purpose gives us a reason to live. Focusing on *living* our passion rather than on dying of cancer or disease brings us back to our true self, which rebuilds the immune system and creates health. If we are focusing on what we are really passionate about in life and truly living life with passion, we are filling our bodies with the energy that facilitates healing. Whereas, *if we have no passion for life and focus on our disease, it is the disease that grows instead of our passion.*

I believe that most people die of cancer and disease because they had just given up on life. They felt that they had nothing to live for. Their children were grown, or their spouse had left, or they hated their job and their life had lost its meaning. They had lost their life's purpose—their passion—and had no zest for life. As important as it is being a parent, spouse, or having a career, we all have a deeper life's purpose beyond that—a mission that is our part in helping to make the world a better place and that actualizes our potential. And *it is of the utmost importance to find our passion for life in healing disease.*

Where is *your* passion hiding? You will benefit greatly from asking yourself that question daily. To find your passion, ask yourself the deeper questions: What is my purpose in life? Why am I here? Who am I? What do I really want to be and do during my lifetime? It helps to keep a journal and allow whatever passes through your mind to be written down. Start with the statement, "What I like to do most is _____." Jot down anything that your hand pulls you to write. It does not have to make sense; keep on writing automatically. Even if nothing comes up for you to write in the beginning, the more you practice doing this, the more likely that one day something *will* come to you, and you will suddenly start feeling excited.

Some of my students discover that their passion for life is renewed when they volunteer their time for a good cause. Others have joined Big Brother or Big Sister to help youngsters feel loved. Some have joined Toastmasters and have found that they have a talent for speaking in front of people and have gone on to become professional speakers. I discovered that I loved volunteering my time at writers' conferences and felt energized meeting so many talented writers, agents, and publishers.

Many people over the age of 60 have started new ventures such as learning a new language, which also sharpens the mind. Others take up painting, singing, dancing, swimming with dolphins, skating, tennis, writing books, making documentary or feature films, acting, or whatever feeds their passion.

Sometimes cancer or another disease is a solution to problems that we see no other way out of. It brings to our attention the deeper issues of life that we have not been willing to address, those that have taken us away from our life's purpose. I now see that my own cancer saved my life. I thought that I had everything. I was very successful as a psychologist. I was earning lots of money. I had many friends. It looked like I had everything anyone could wish for. Yet I remember feeling a yearning to be in alignment with my true purpose in life. *There was an emptiness that I did not understand.* I wanted to feel closer to my true self and the pure love that I had felt inside on a number of occasions. My ex-husband did not believe in God, so I had shut down the spiritual part of me to please him.

I loved connecting with spiritual people who cared about the world, about the earth, and who were active in helping heal humanity in real and meaningful ways. Even though my soul was yearning to feel the deep love of the Divine and yearning to do my part alongside these people, my busy life did not allow time for that. I had disconnected from my true self and my passion. *I was dying inside without knowing it.* The solution came in the form of cancer. My body was telling me, "If you don't live the life you want to live, then I am checking out on you." That woke me up.

Finding my passion for life gave me a renewed sense of a reason to live. While practicing the exercises in this book when I was healing from cancer, I would get glimpses of a yearning to erase sickness, pain, and suffering from humanity. The more I focused on my passion rather than on cancer, the more I felt my true self emerge. Being and living who I really am has helped rebuild my immune system and has created radiant health in my body.

My passion is constantly unfolding. The first glimpses of my life purpose have become even more potent. Now I know that my greatest passion is to help heal the pain and sickness that I see all around me everywhere in the world that I go. *When I align myself with this passion, I feel new energy pouring throughout my body.* I am filled with such excitement and enthusiasm to help make this happen. And it is such fun.

I am grateful for my body's message of love. Cancer has been a blessing in disguise. It has given me a life of freedom and joy. Before cancer, I would not have allowed myself to have this much fun without feeling guilty. I would have thought it was selfish to have fun the way that my heart wanted. Now, I get to feel the connection of divine love and spend time with the spiritual people that I love who are also fulfilling their soul's craving by living their passion and helping humanity, each in their own way.

For those who say, "It's too late. I'm too old to find my passion or my life's purpose. I've lived my life and now it's over," I remind you of what Richard Bach said in his best-selling book, *Illusions*—that if you are still alive, you have not completed your purpose. I am now in my 60s—the age when others are thinking of retiring—and I feel I am just getting started. I'm just beginning my life's purpose. I want to live to a ripe old age—over 120—to experiment with all I have learned to the fullest. As I focus on my passion of helping to erase sickness, a return to youthfulness seems to be a natural by-product of the renewed energy I feel. I envision myself at age 120, looking and feeling as healthy and young as I look now. When I am in my passion, I feel ageless, and often people take me to be a lot younger than I am.

When challenging disease, it is important to focus on goals that excite your imagination. It doesn't matter if you think it is real or not. Many geniuses were ridiculed when new inspiring ideas appeared to them. One hundred years ago, if you told someone that there will one day be winged vehicles that could lift up and fly in the air, they would probably think you were crazy. A realistic goal that helped me and my students heal is to see yourself playing with your grandchildren and watching them grow up. Visualize yourself loving, nurturing, and guiding them to understand how wonderful they are, helping them to feel secure and safe. The desire to stay alive to be a part of their lives helps the body heal itself.

Envision your goals achieved, your books published, your talents improving, and yourself achieving new possibilities. See yourself with family and friends celebrating holidays together, visiting new countries you have never been to before, finding new adventures, swimming with dolphins, and doing everything you have always wanted to do. Be creative, be inventive, be courageous, and allow your imagination to flow. Write the images that inspire you in your journal, whenever they come to you.

When I felt that I was dying, my close friend helped me create a colorful collage of the goals I wanted to achieve in the future. I hung it on the refrigerator door and looked at it daily. I have achieved all those goals and a lot more that I did not think of at that time.

Make a collage of your dreams. Cut images that appeal to you from magazines and paste them together on a sheet of poster paper. Hang it in a place where you will see it on a daily basis. Remember how Jacob's sheep gave birth to spotted babies? Use your imagination to create collages of your wildest dreams. Don't judge them as impossible. Enjoy the images they produce. Imagine each time you look at it that you have achieved these goals and feel the sensations of joy of having it all. Watch the way your body responds, releasing chemicals that strengthen and heal your body.

New visions may appear to you from time to time as you focus on your heart's bliss and living your passion. I suggest you write them down as they show up. That's how new inventions have appeared in our lives.

Edison envisioned the possibility of having electricity. It was a wild vision that met with a lot of ridicule and skepticism and was discarded as crazy. Edison failed countless times before he finally succeeded. Can you imagine what life was like without electricity—no computers, no radio, no television, no DVD players, no washers or dryers, stoves, heaters, hairdryers, or any of the electric appliances we now take for granted, and no light at the flip of a switch when we walk into a room? All these things that are now such an important part of our lives have only come about in the last hundred years because one man had the courage to follow his visions. Edison was asked by a reporter, "You failed a thousand times, why didn't you give up?"

He responded, "I never failed once. I just did not do it the right way. Each time was a success because what you call failure just showed me what does not work."

Your body shows you what does not work when you get sick. Let your heart and passion show you what *does* work so you can create a healthy, vital, joyful, and passionate life.

Exercise for Creating Bliss and Finding Your Passion

To create bliss and find your passion, do the following seven steps: (You may wish to close your eyes so that you are more deeply focused on what you are doing.)

1. Focus your attention on your heart, in the center of your chest. Imagine that your heart is like a huge lung. As you inhale,

expand the size of your heart and as you exhale, squeeze any stagnant energy out while saying the sound *haaaaaaaaa*. Do this three times.

2. Imagine any situations in your life that are stressful. Feel them in your heart as you convert the energy they produce into love. Smile to your heart and imagine feeling it smiling back to you.

3. Continue doing this exercise with each organ and each part of your body. (It would be helpful to get an anatomy book and become familiar with the size, shape, and the location of each part of the body you are working on.)

    a. Do the same with your lungs three times. Exchange smiles with your lungs on either side of your heart.

    b. Do the same with your liver, located at the right side of your body beneath the ribcage.

    c. Do the same with your kidneys, located at the small of your back, the size of small fists.

    d. Do the same with your stomach, located at the left side of your body under your ribcage.

    e. Do the same with your spleen, located beside your stomach.

    f. Do the same with your pancreas, located underneath your stomach.

    g. Do the same with your gallbladder located under your liver.

    h. Do the same with your adrenal glands, sitting on top of your kidneys.

    i. Do the same with your bladder, located in the lower abdomen.

    j. Do the same with your sexual organs. (For women, the ovaries located at the sides of the lower abdomen. For men, the testicles.)

    k. Do the same with your thymus gland, located above the heart.

    l. Do the same with your thyroid gland, located in the throat.

    m. Do the same with your brain and the midbrain.

    n. Do the same with your face, and your hair.

o. Do the same with your bones.

p. Do the same with your hands.

q. And do the same with your feet.

You may do it in any order you wish, whatever part of the body shows up for you to focus on.

4. Notice the sensations in your body change as you do it. Continue until you feel joy and bliss.

5. Ask your heart, "What is your passion? What would you enjoy doing today that will be nurturing to you?" Wait quietly for a response.

6. Ask your heart again, "What would you enjoy doing if all your needs were taken care of? If you had all the money you wish and all the support you need, what would you do with your life?" Wait quietly for a response.

You don't have to try to think of a response. The response will show up at the right time. It may come in unexpected ways. The universe has unusual ways of expressing itself. You may meet a friend who tells you something and your heart responds with a sensation that says, "Yes, that's what would nurture me and give me joy to do." For example, you may hear someone talking about Oprah Winfrey's talk show and happen to watch that day when the theme is focused on finding your passion. Or you may see a hawk flying high overhead and feel a yearning to go for a walk in nature.

7. Make a decision to plan to do it. *Follow the intuitive calling that is guiding you from within.* Take a walk in nature as soon as you can. You may notice that new ideas emerge while connecting with the beauty of nature. Plan to act according to the ideas you receive and decide when you will be taking that action.

Creating a Healthy Life

Once you have begun focusing on your life's passion, you may want to use the following exercise to accelerate living your life's purpose and creating a healthy life. I have been using this technique for some time to achieve my life goals as well as to heal from cancer. I was often amazed at the speed at which my desires were achieved. I discovered that the desires that are in alignment with the highest good show up in my life as soon as I let go of my resistance to feeling worthy of having them.

A key to breaking through your resistance to deserving being healed is to use the phrase, "I am now willing..." For instance, "I am now willing to be in good health. I open to believing that I deserve it. I am now willing to own my power to be fulfilled, happy, energetic, healthy, and abundant. I open my cells to the Divine love flowing within my bones in harmony and bliss. I release chemicals and hormones from my brain sending messages of feeling safe, protected, loved, loving, and happy. I feel sincere reverence for my immune system and the natural healing mechanism built within my body. My body knows how to heal itself. I surrender to the Divine energy of love, God's purest Divine love, and my highest good within me."

The benefits of practicing this exercise include freedom from disease, the ability to respond with calm and ease to stressful situations, and having your heart's desires come true. An example is that I wanted to heal from cancer and live by the sea. For over 40 years, I have lived in places other than by the ocean. I thought I was kidding myself that I could find a way to live the life of my dreams. After doing this exercise on a regular basis, I now live in Hawaii, cancer free for more than seven years, just steps from the ocean. All day and all night, the sound of the waves soothe me, nurture me and fill me with delight.

This exercise is based on what I learned from teachers, such as Deepak Chopra and Master Haidakhan Babaji.

Exercise to Create a Healthy Life

To create a healthy life, do the following five steps:

1. Write down your vision, your passion, your purpose in life. Imagine what you would do when you have everything you have ever wanted; more money than you could possibly spend; and as much love, friendship, and assistance as you wish. Pay attention to your true desires. Describe your goals to yourself in as much detail as possible. Also, write down your desired state of health as if it were already achieved. For example, "My cells are radiating with health; any diseased cells are dissolved rapidly as new healthy cells emerge."

2. Imagine your goals are already achieved. Feel the vibrations of love, joy, and peace radiating with light in your body. *When we vibrate with these high energies, we magnetize what we are imaging to materialize in our lives.*

3. To know that you are worthy to receive the desired outcome, repeat over and over deep in your heart and mind: "I give myself permission to allow abundance of all good health, specifically _____ (fill in the gap of what it is you desire) into my life, for the highest good of everything and everyone, including me."

4. A master teacher taught me: "Everything can be achieved through the constant repetition of words that vibrate with the purest love. It is a powerful mind tool."

As I repeated the words "purest Divine love" (*Om Namaha Shivaya* in Sanskrit) constantly to myself, my mind calmed down, and I felt as though I was resting in the purest of love. I still repeat those words. I have been practicing this exercise for many years, sometimes with astounding results. It has not only helped me achieve my desires, I believe it has saved my life several times. When I was feeling most desperate, I realized that I had forgotten to repeat those words and remembered that everything can be achieved by repeating them. I was intrigued to discover that just *remembering* to repeat those words instantly ignited my hope and inspired me to know that I can heal.

Some people find that repeating the name of God works well for them. Choose a word or phrase that, when you repeat it, makes you feel love in your heart. For example, "I repeat with sincerity the highest vibration of pure love that heals all that needs to be healed within me and creates a new healthy life."

5. Release your desires to your wise higher self, a higher power, God, or the universe. Be neutral, unattached to the results, feeling peaceful. Allow your higher self to take over and bring into your life the desires that are for your greatest good. It will be delivered to you when the time is right. That has been my experience. *As we believe, we create.* Watch your world: What have you believed and created? As you strengthen your ability to create healthy, joyful beliefs and images, your world will "outpicture" them.

Practice this exercise daily, once a day for several minutes until you achieve your goal. Then, choose a new goal. However, keep on repeating your chosen words in the back of your mind 24 hours a day or as often as you remember. I hummed the words to melodies I developed or to any music I heard. You can tell your subconscious mind to keep on repeating those words while talking, working, or sleeping.

A word of caution: Use this exercise only for positive goals, such as improving your health, your life, and the lives of those around you. If you are angry or hurt and wish for revenge, you may harm yourself in the process of wishing for something bad to happen to those you are angry with. *The feelings of revenge are toxic; the body releases these feelings as chemicals that cause sickness.* Evaporate feelings of revenge, anger, and resentment into feelings of forgiveness, compassion, and love. *You* benefit the most from the vibrations of these positive qualities. Let the universe, the law of cause and effect, or God take care of those people you perceive have hurt you. Believe that justice always prevails; we may not always know the how, and it isn't important. What is important is for your body to feel good and maintain radiant health.

Chapter 12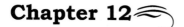

Step Nine: Creating a Healing Environment to Reverse or Prevent Disease

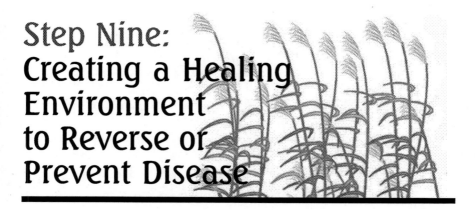

Seven-year-old Tim lived with a sense of insecurity and low self-esteem. After he lost all his hair during chemotherapy, he felt ashamed of his bald head, which only added to his low opinion of himself. He covered up that shame by constantly lying, exaggerating, and picking fights with his younger sister. He was also having problems at school.

"Why do young children, even babies, get cancer?" asked his mother, Lisa. "Surely they haven't yet developed unhealthy thought patterns."

"Children are very open, vulnerable, and sensitive," I replied. "They can feel the emotions created by their parents' thought patterns very easily."

"Really?" Lisa asked.

"Those vibrations are contagious," I continued. "Even though the parents may not have cancer, their child is exposed to the combination of inherited toxic thought patterns of both parents. The child's body reflects those patterns."

Lisa responded, "Now I remember reading about a scientific study that showed even babies in the womb are affected by the mother's emotions during pregnancy."

"That's right. The good news is that parents can help their children heal the emotional problems and disease that result from these toxic attitudes." I recommended that the family form their own healing circle support group to teach Tim self-healing techniques.

While practicing the exercises, the parents began to identify their own inherited toxic thought patterns. Lisa said, "My husband and I discovered that we also exaggerate and lie and so did our parents. Now we understand that this need was a result of our own feeling of being unloved growing up. We realized that our subconscious beliefs that we weren't good enough prompted us to treat Tim in a way that also made him feel not good enough. It makes sense why Tim lied to try to impress others."

Lisa admitted, "I noticed that I hadn't been able to look Tim in the eye. That upset me. I find it easier to love my daughter than to love Tim. That must hurt his feelings. He can see it in my eyes." A few weeks later Lisa commented, "The more we have been practicing these exercises, the more I am becoming aware of Tim's positive qualities and the more love I feel for him. I can now look into his eyes with love."

Her husband, Henry, added, "It was Tim who wanted us to tell him that we love him. We immediately started doing that. Focusing on our decision to appreciate and love each other and ourselves makes it easier to give and receive love. It's amazing how good that makes us feel."

Tim's grades improved, his need to lie diminished, and his relationship with his sister improved. As the family continued doing the exercises regularly, Tim slowly regained his health. Tim's hair grew back along with his confidence that he would not have a recurrence.

That was more than 20 years ago. Tim is now happily married with children of his own and is president of his own company.

Research has shown that people who feel supported and cared for do much better healing from cancer and other diseases than those who do not have support. Therefore, *connecting with encouraging, nurturing, supportive people on a regular basis is crucial to your healing*. However, current statistics reveal that more than a third of the people diagnosed with cancer and other diseases do not have a support system.

I believe that if I had nurturing, nourishing, and spiritually supportive people to connect with regularly, I would not have gotten cancer. At the time, I did not know that was what I needed. Had I known, I would have searched out or created that kind of support circle. Now, that support is an integral part of my life and health.

I don't mean just any kind of support, because sometimes what is called support can actually be debilitating—even from good-intentioned family, friends, and support groups. Unfortunately, the only kinds of groups available are the standard cancer support groups, *which focus on illness rather than on health, healing, and prevention.*

Here is the common feedback I receive from my students about these groups:

"I attended two different cancer support groups, and they both were really grim. Some kindness and caring, but absolutely no positive encouragement that it was possible to heal instead of die. They were just holding each other together until they died."

"When I attended some of these groups, I became so depressed. I felt hopeless."

"Witnessing others' pain, losing close friends who don't make it and die, imprinted deep attitudes of fear and desperation within me."

I recently spoke with a cancer client, a teacher from Los Angeles, who said:

"The cancer support group I was attending was too depressing. *I would come back home feeling worse.*"

What We Hear Affects Us

When we challenge cancer or any disease, we are more open and vulnerable to what we hear. Notice when someone says something to you, how your mind repeats it over and over many times, like a tape recorder that automatically keeps rewinding and replaying the same thing. Sometimes these thoughts stay with you for several days. It takes a lot of energy to disregard them and not be affected if the messages are negative and harmful.

After my third bout with cancer—even though I had gathered a lot of wisdom and was beginning to practice the self-healing techniques in this book—doubts would creep in unnoticed. I would do great when I was alone without interaction with my family. But as soon as I felt good and strong, I would start reconnecting with family and friends. However, *their fears and doubts were so contagious that I would start feeling sick again.*

I remember how sick I would feel when I heard horror stories of people dying from cancer. It affected me so badly that my strange symptoms intensified immediately, and my tumor grew rapidly. It took me a long time to realize this connection. I just thought that cancer was back again and that it had nothing to do with the outside world. Every little cold, new pain, or tiredness I felt made me panicky that cancer had returned. I had little or no support to maintain my new knowing and healing decisions.

I often heard remarks from well-meaning friends and relatives, such as "You are fooling yourself, you must go to the hospital." These remarks would play over and over in my mind until my immune system weakened, and my symptoms confirmed that cancer had spread. In retrospect, that was the most difficult part in healing myself. *I nearly died before I became aware of what was happening.*

On one occasion a relative of mine came to visit and said, "You have a lot of nerve not listening to the doctors and not doing chemotherapy. Who do you think you are?" A part of me knew that she did not understand the power of self-healing, but I still felt frightened because I was exploring new territory that I was not yet sure of myself. (This relative recently died from a disease where for years she had been following the doctor's orders and taking all kinds of medications to treat it.)

When I followed my heart's guidance and would leave home to be in a more positive atmosphere, my body responded almost immediately. I would feel better and hopeful that I could heal myself. As soon as I returned home, however, my body would start decaying in front of my eyes. Because I was not as aware in those days as I am now, I didn't see the connection.

"Hey, my family loves me," I thought to myself. "Why would I get sick again being with them?" It did not make sense. I loved them and wanted to be with them. What I didn't realize was that they were not capable of nurturing my self-healing decisions because they were caught in their own fears. All they knew was the medical route, and they believed that cancer was death. Therefore, they could not help being trapped in thoughts of terror.

Others' toxic thought patterns affect us too. They don't even have to say anything; we feel their thoughts inside us in our subconscious, which affects us. To most people, even the very mention of the word "cancer" creates panic. Many people never mention this word. My friend said, "Sarah passed away." "What did she die from?" I asked. She just nodded her head with a serious expression on her face. She didn't want to even say the word "cancer."

Studies in family therapy have shown that when hospitalized mental patients became better after therapy, they would be discharged as "improved." However, after a period of time being back at home, having to deal with the same thought patterns that made them sick, they would lose whatever ground they'd gained and be hospitalized again. From my experience, this is also true with cancer or any disease.

For example, even people who have attended my workshops have regressed after returning home. They often say, "I felt so wonderful after I attended your workshop, but a few weeks later I crashed and started feeling miserable again." What happens during the workshop is that they focus on the truth of their deeper true self, which is joy, love, peace, radiant health, and their full potential, which naturally makes them feel good. As soon as people go back home where there may not be support and understanding of these healing principles, they hear the old negative attitudes, and it affects them.

At the time when I was so weak and traumatized with fear of possibly dying a horrible death any day, even watching television affected me. I would start feeling nauseous for no apparent reason. What we see on television is so filled with negative images that it affects our bodies.

I rarely watch television now—only *Oprah* and movies that are entertaining, uplifting, and make me laugh. Laughter is very healing. It releases chemicals that give us a euphoric high that strengthens the immune system.

For example, Norman Cousins, longtime editor of *The Saturday Review* magazine who was given six months to live by his doctors, decided that he wanted to enjoy his life for those few months. He checked into a hotel room and watched funny movies all day. He told his friends that he just wanted to laugh and asked them not to visit him unless they were going to tell him jokes. He laughed so much that he got well. He lived for many more years and went on to write a number of books, including *Anatomy of an Illness* and *Head First: The Biology of Hope and the Healing Power of the Human Spirit*, and to lecture worldwide.

Most people cannot afford to check into a hotel room or travel to a healing resort to be in a supportive, uplifting environment that empowers us to heal. The next best thing is to connect with a truly healing support group on a regular basis that supports us to *heal*.

Just as negative words can debilitate us and make us sick, on the other hand when we hear words that support and encourage the notion that we *can* heal, we are reminded that we have the ability to heal ourselves. And then that is what buzzes in our heads over and over many times each day. Usually it is not always possible for us to be surrounded by enlightened people who are inspiring and supportive. That's why joining or forming a nurturing, supportive healing group is so vital—especially one that reminds you of what is possible after you have forgotten or become discouraged. When you are feeling down, it can boost your spirits and energy, lift you up, and put you back on track for healing.

The kind of support I'm talking about uplifts you so that you feel encouraged and empowered to do whatever you need to heal. *The support that healing groups can provide is not only life saving, but an integral part of the healing process.* With the encouragement and support of others who are developing similar thought patterns, it is much easier to make the necessary changes to reverse or prevent disease. Your consciousness will be filled with strong, healthy, healing decisions. Then, notice how they repeat themselves in your thoughts throughout the week.

Because the current cancer support groups don't provide tools that show you how to heal yourself, obviously these groups don't work if you are interested in regaining your health. What is really needed is a focus on healing and living rather than on disease and dying. It has been proven that support groups help cancer patients survive longer. In my eyes, longer is not acceptable when cancer can be reversed for good. Because reversal or prevention is possible—as my clients, students, and I have demonstrated—then it would be foolish to settle for a few more years of poor-quality life when you can enjoy life in radiant health until a ripe old age.

If you would like to be part of a Healing Circle support group, go to my Website: *www.youheal.com*. You will find a complete program, "Healing and Prevention Support Program for Patients, Loved Ones, Caregivers, and Healthcare Professionals." This system gives you in-depth guidance on how to continue your growth with the support of a powerful healing environment.

How fast are you willing to have health and a wonderful life? How long do you want to feel unhealthy and not good enough? One of the most powerful steps you can take on your journey back to health is to create a healing environment to reverse your disease. It is the finest gift you can give yourself to support your healing.

Chapter 13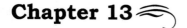

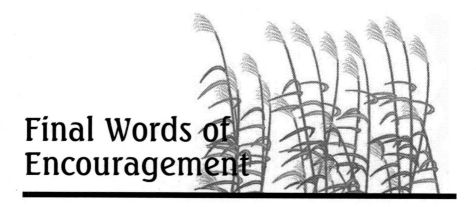

Final Words of Encouragement

In March 1994, my doctor told me my cancerous breast tumor had shrunk to half its size. I felt deep joy. I knew I was on the right track and that I would heal. I continued practicing my Daily Healing Routine three times a day.

There were days, however, when doubts would creep in. I might have spoken with someone whose cancer had spread and become discouraged. My doctor's words of warning would suddenly appear in my mind, "Yes, it is cancer and you must go to the hospital immediately."

"But the tumor has shrunk," I would remind myself. However, when doubts came in, my ability to visualize diminished, and my healing practice did not do anything for me. I would tell myself,

> "Protect your energy. Speak with someone who loves you and supports your self-healing work. Give yourself permission to avoid reading newspapers or watching television programs that upset you. Stay away from well-meaning people who make you doubt your ability to heal yourself. Go within, and connect with the wisdom of your inner guidance. Slow down, and enjoy just being and breathing. Do what gives you joy to do right now. Remember that others have done it, and so can you."

I canceled all outside activities and sat quietly with myself. It was not easy at first. From time to time, I felt the terrible pain of loneliness. I remembered one of my relatives telling me, "You can go crazy being alone." I stayed with the pain, breathing into it, and feeling it completely. I gave myself permission to cry and feel all my emotions fully. I took time to rest and stay in bed.

I felt guilty for doing what my mind thought of as nothing. Thoughts of, "You should do this and you should do that," constantly interfered with my trying to relax and let go. I challenged those impulses that ordered me to do, do, do. I told myself, "If you die, what good are all those things you feel that you must do rather than rest?"

The more I rested and spent time alone in silence, the more my energy grew and soon my joy reappeared. When I once again felt joy, the self-healing work became more powerful, and my body started regaining vitality and strength.

As soon as I was feeling wonderful again, I forgot how desperate and hopeless I'd felt only a few days before. I started taking on new projects, meeting with people, interacting with the outside world—and I would go back into "overwhelm." My energy would drain once more.

I had to train myself to become deeply in tune with the signs my body was giving me. A slight tension would tell me: "Stop, go back to taking it easy before your energy is drained again." It was a challenge because I was treading on new territory. There was no one to show me the way.

As I learned to focus on protecting my energy, my body regained radiant health. Eight months later, my doctor confirmed that my cancer was gone.

Creating Radiant Health

If you don't see results right away, don't be discouraged or forget to practice these exercises. It took a long time to create your disease. And it may take time to reverse it. Nothing is possible without patience. Imagine you are in timelessness. Slow down, do less. More is not better. On the path to health, doing less works best.

If you are feeling discouraged, it is a sign that you are in overwhelm. You are trying too hard, doing too much. Breathe and relax. Simplify your life. Give up everything that is not empowering and supporting you on your road to health. Choose the path of least effort. Do something joyful to perk up your energy. Go for a walk, have a massage, sit in a Jacuzzi, watch a funny movie, go shopping, or whatever lifts your spirit.

When resistance shows up anywhere in my body, this is the exercise I do. In my mind's eye, I open it up and wash it with the liquid love from my heart. When I imagine opening it up, I often see images of destructive fire burning until the liquid of pure love is poured over it, and the resistance disappears. Repeating the name of a higher power or a statement of focused intention while placing my attention on that area seems to help me understand the message my body is giving me. The message is often, "Breathe, slow down, connect with the feeling of joy inside." There is nothing more important to creating health than feeling wonderful inside.

Other times I imagine talking to that part of me that is frightened, which could be old patterns from childhood. I take that little girl who was afraid and hug her and fill her heart with love. I tell her that she is good and encourage her to tell me all she is feeling. I may hear her say, "There is so much to do and I don't know how to do it all." I then respond, "I am willing to place my trust in my wise self to guide me what to do next with ease, joy, and laughter." When I repeat this statement sincerely, with reverence, I realign myself with my wise self, and I find myself being in the flow once more. Everything gets handled efficiently and effortlessly.

Ask for help from a higher power or your spiritual source. Ask to be guided. Listen and wait quietly for signs from your inner wisdom. Choose one simple new attitude to practice whenever you remember. You may wish to try this phrase: "I can rest my mind and nurture my confidence in my ability to learn to heal myself. I have learned to do many things, and, in time, I will master this too."

Don't feel like you have to do all the exercises every day. The Daily Healing Routine is important to do on a daily basis. Then practice the exercise of your choice that you feel will help you the most. Some exercises may not be necessary for you to do right now. The exercises are just guidelines to help you find your own way to what will heal not only your body, but also your life. Learn to trust your wisdom to guide you to what images would be most helpful to you and strengthen the connection with your true self. You can mix and match sections or sentences from any exercise and create your own version of what you wish to practice or what would serve you best. With practice and time, you will excel in these exercises and create radiant health.

I have given you the program that enabled me to heal myself of breast cancer during the third and worst occurrence and return to radiant health—without medical intervention. The information and exercises in this book have shown you that you also have the ability to erase pain, suffering, and disease from your life.

There is one last story I would like to share with you, another testimonial to the power of self-healing when you are challenging cancer and other life-threatening diseases.

In 1987, Beverly was only in her 30s when she was diagnosed with renal cell carcinoma (kidney cancer). She underwent surgery to remove her right kidney and remained cancer-free for 14 years. But in 2001, the cancer had metastisized to her pancreas. She underwent a Whipple procedure, which is the surgical removal of the pancreas, gall bladder, spleen, duodenum, and part of the stomach.

Recovery from this procedure is extremely difficult, and it took Beverly seven months to feel somewhat normal. She also suffered from depression during most of her recovery. When the follow-up MRI revealed metastatic renal cells on her liver, she and her husband, Elliot, were not sure what to do. They felt a looming sense of hopelessness.

In November 2002 Beverly went to the City of Hope Cancer Center in California for a series of IL2 treatments. In this form of chemotherapy, the patient is given high doses of a drug that boosts the white cell count, hopefully to kill the cancer. It is a very harsh treatment—patients have to remain in the intensive-care ward completely bedridden for one week. They go home for two weeks and then return for another session. The side effects are much worse than from normal chemo.

Her follow-up MRI showed that the tumors had not only increased in size but also in number. There was no reason to continue the treatment. Beverly was not given any other treatment options by her medical team. She felt lost and all alone in her battle.

Beverly then tried a high-bolus vitamin C therapy, but the cost was a staggering $10,000 a month. She used the treatment for about three months, then told her doctor that she could no longer afford it. The doctor said he was unable to reduce the price. That was her very last chance...or so she thought.

Beverly began reading inspirational books by Dr. Wayne Dyer. They opened her mind to many possibilities. When her husband wrote to the author explaining her situation, Dr. Dyer wrote back and told him about an upcoming healing seminar in Maui, given by Dr. Shivani Goodman.

"Shivani's exercises really work," he added.

Beverly attented the seminar with her husband and eagerly learned to perform the healing techniques.

Within two months after her return home—after faithfully following the methods explained in this book—Beverly had another MRI. It showed that the tumors had not only decreased in numbers, but the larger ones were starting to die from the center.

Beverly continues to get stronger and healthier every day.

Self-healing is a journey. Allow yourself the time to reach your destination and be patient with yourself along the way. Focus on your heart's desire, and do what brings you joy. Refer daily to the nine steps on the following page to ensure you are doing what is needed to successfully reach your goal.

Remember, others have done it, and so can you!

❦ THE 9 STEPS ❧

1. Make a Decision to Be Well
Decide to live in radiant health.

2. Heal Your Emotional Pain
*Release bad feelings and
develop new healthy feelings.*

3. Heal Your Toxic Attitudes
*Find the unhealthy attitudes that caused
disease and make new healing decisions.*

4. Practice the Daily Healing Routine
*Relax deeply, self-heal, affirm healing
decisions, and consult the wise self within.*

5. Call on the Doctor Within
*Use the wisdom within you to heal disease
and strengthen the immune system.*

6. Use Your Doubt to Create Certainty
*Put doubt in your doubts
to create what you want.*

7. Use Spiritual Energy
to Enhance Your Healing
*Connect to your essence
to access the love that heals.*

8. Follow Your Heart's Bliss
and Live With Passion
*Listen to the voice of your heart
and create a healthy, fulfilling life.*

9. Create a Healing Environment
*Surround yourself with a circle of
encouragement to support your recovery.*

Appendix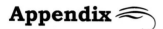

Changing Toxic Attitudes to Healing Decisions

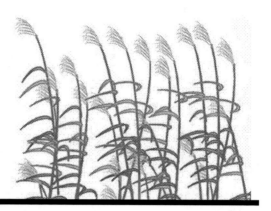

When working with clients challenging cancer and other diseases, I have found that there are common subconscious toxic attitudes. Following are some of the most prevalent ones that can help you pinpoint the attitudes that need to be changed within you. Opposite the self-sabotaging attitude, I have placed an example of a new healing decision to show you how you can create healing decisions out of your own toxic beliefs.

To locate your own toxic attitudes, pay attention to when you feel afraid, upset, or anxious. Usually the emotions emerge more fully at night. Identify and write down your toxic attitudes, and change them to healing decisions. Make copies and carry one with you wherever you go. Anytime you start feeling upset, take out a copy and read both the toxic and healing decisions. You will notice that by reading the toxic decisions that produced the painful emotions, there is a discharge—almost like a zap of static electricity—and the emotions usually calm down.

Notice that when you read the healing decisions, which are healthy and empowering to focus on, pleasant sensations start flowing through you. In addition to placing a copy of the list in your purse or pocket and carrying it with you everywhere you go, practice the new healing decisions after deep relaxation as directed in the Healing Decisions section of Chapters 6 and 7.

My understanding is that the toxic decisions are in our collective unconscious, inherited from our ancestors. The healing decisions are in our superconscious mind, our true self. We can tap into that part of us and convince our subconscious minds to trust and believe in them. They are good for us and can be planted deep into the subconscious by practicing them daily, three times a day. We can choose to feel good while we watch them grow into beautiful fruit trees that feed us all.

If you find it difficult to identify your toxic attitudes, use some of the following examples to get you started. Begin by working on the ones that are the most toxic and are interfering with your life. You may then wish to refine them by identifying your own that are of particular issue in your personal life.

Notice that the toxic decisions in the first section are written in the past tense. This may help you open to the fresh and new in the here and now.

RELATIONSHIP TO SELF AND OTHERS

Toxic Attitudes	Healing Decisions
1. Until now, I felt ashamed of my existence. I felt guilty if I perceived myself to be imperfect. I thought that I had to be perfect and do everything perfectly in order to survive.	1. It is safe to enjoy my life. I am a fallible human being like all other human beings—no more, no less, and what we perceive as fallible is transitory. I now see my imperfections as a perfect opportunity for growth.
2. It is terrible to be fallible; I hated it. I believed that others disapproved of me and, therefore, I must disapprove of myself. The more I approve of myself, the more others approve of me.	2. It is wonderful to be fallible. The more I love it, the more it changes. My true nature grows. The more I approve of myself, the more others approve of me. And my health grows.
3. Until now I felt unworthy of love because I showed off and felt ashamed of myself.	3. I open my heart to know that I am worthy of love. I am changing what is changeable according to my guidance.

4. I thought it was shameful and a weakness to be good.

4. It may or may not be desirable to be good. I trust my inner knowing to guide me.

5. I believed I should have no needs.

5. Everyone has needs, and so do I.

6. I decided that when I love, I should receive love in return—that it is humiliating and painful to love and not feel loved back.

6. It is healthy and safe to love. Whether others love me is a reflection of how much they love themselves.

7. I need to be loved by others in order to love myself. If others don't show me their love I will die feeling abandoned, rejected, and unwanted.

7. I may or may not receive love and I can always depend on the love of my true self or a higher power to satisfy my needs. I can choose to feel love for myself and others. When I love others, I benefit by feeling the vibrations of love whether they love me or not.

8. I decided that if I love deeply, I will be made fun of and would feel hurt.

8. I may or may not be made fun of for loving deeply, but how I respond inside is up to me. I always allow myself to feel comfortable now.

9. I decided that I must feel afraid of being attacked for feeling loved by others. They will feel jealous, find something wrong with me to put me down.

9. I may or may not be attacked for being loved, and I am taking care of myself in all circumstances, according to my own inner guidance.

10. I decided to believe that it is either you or me. If someone else is bright, pretty, or rich, then I must be stupid, ugly, or poor.

10. It is both you *and* me. Others may be bright, prett,y and rich and, so am I. They may or may not be more or better than me, and I feel good either way.

11. I accepted the decision that I must be nice or else I will be disliked and hurt by others.

11. I have a choice of being nice or not nice as I wish. I can always be authentic to my real self.

12. I decided to accept the decision that I had to say and do the right thing to make the right impression on others.

12. When I feel free to feel good and be who I really am, I make the best impression.

13. When I felt manipulated by people, I chose to feel bad, inferior, small, and humiliated.

13. People don't manipulate me. I respond to people's interactions, and I choose healthy, calm responses.

14. It may not be safe to tell the truth.

14. The truth is freeing, and I can learn to discern when it is safe to be open and sensitively honest and when it is okay to be silent.

15. I chose to believe that it was dangerous to be honest, that people would take advantage of me and hurt me.

15. It is important to be sensitively honest; people may still respond in undesirable ways. I am taking care of myself.

16. I decided that I must protect my brothers and sisters even if they were vicious.

16. My brothers and sisters can protect themselves. They may or may not be vicious, and I am taking care of myself.

17. I chose to believe that I had to accept people's thoughts and projections on me as valid and invalidate my knowing.

17. People's thoughts and projections may or may not be valid. It is their business, not mine. I am free to take care of my business and respond as I see fit.

18. Everything that goes wrong anywhere in the world I believed to be my fault.

18. I am a fallible human being, no more, no less. It's okay to just be.

19. I thought that I had to sacrifice myself in order to protect and help others.

19. I can protect others better by staying alive if protecting and helping others is what I want to do.

20. I decided that whatever I do is sometimes not okay. It may not be perfect, and I had to worry constantly about others' responses.

20. I always do the best I can. People may respond in agreeable or disagreeable ways, and I choose to feel comfortable either way.

21. War is terrifying. They may kill me or my family.

21. What's supposed to happen will happen. I am alive now, and I can choose to enjoy feeling alive.

22. I may die a horrible and torturous death.

22. I can choose to believe that I will die a natural death with a sense of completion, fulfillment, and satisfaction, when I am sure that I have finished my life's work on earth.

In the sections that follow, the toxic statements are written in the present tense. See which tense works best for you to identify your own toxic decisions. If you wish, you may then change the toxic decisions to the past tense.

CULTURAL INFLUENCES

1. I must believe what society tells me to believe and build my life according to others' thoughts and opinions.

1. I take away my reality that I built on false premises and give myself a new reality. I forgive myself for building my life on the thoughts and opinions of others that are based on faulty thinking. I am now willing to own the truth and allow the purest and highest reality into my life. Love is very healing. I open my heart to feel the healing love deep inside. I choose my thoughts and my life to reflect this love.

FEAR OF FAILURE OR SUCCESS

1. I have to feel pain when I don't do things the right way.

1. I can choose to feel content inside knowing that I always do my best, whether I do things the right way or not. If I do things the wrong way, I can learn from my mistakes, which show me where I can learn and grow.

2. Sometimes I sabotage my success by doing and saying stupid things and then feel embarrassed, uncomfortable, and hate myself.

2. I am now encouraging my knowing that I deserve to be successful. As my awareness grows, I will say and do things that support my success. I can always feel compassion and love for myself, whatever I perceive myself to be saying or doing. The more love I feel for myself, the more I will say and do things that enhance my success.

3. I must be more than I am. If someone is better than me, that means that I am inferior.

3. I am fine as I am. There will always be someone better in certain areas or have certain skills that I don't have. I may be better than someone else in certain areas or have certain skills that others may not have. It is impossible to compare and I can choose to feel good being just as I am. Every person has a unique gift to share with others.

4. Only if I am rich and famous will others respect me and seek me out.

4. I choose to feel wonderful about myself and my life right now. If others seek me out because I am rich and famous, they are not the true friends that I want to be with anyway.

5. I have to understand everything that is happening everywhere or else I will be vulnerable and others will take advantage of me. I am not strong enough to take care of myself.

5. I know what I know and it is okay to not know what I don't know. I can stand up for myself when needed. No one can take advantage of me unless I let them. My strength is growing every day. I can take care of myself.

6. I have to pretend to be strong so that others won't see how frightened I really am. People are like animals; they can sense that I am afraid and manipulate me to their advantage.

6. The more peaceful I am with myself, the less frightened I am. I can practice self-healing exercises every day to be more focused on my true self and seek calm. The more calm I feel, the less frightened I will be. People may or may not behave in desirable ways, and I can take care of myself according to my inner guidance.

7. My body betrayed me. My disease will kill me. I am bound to fail.

7. The more I practice the healing decisions after deep relaxation, the quieter and better I feel. The body's natural healing mechanisms are then triggered, and my body knows how to heal itself. My survival is built within me.

8. If someone is more successful than I am, I think I am a failure or not good enough.

8. I am always good enough as I am. There will always be someone better at something, and I can choose to feel fine.

GUILT

1. I am guilty; I should have known better. I should have chosen to act or say things differently.

1. I have always done the best I could with the awareness, resources, and strength I had at

the time. As my awareness grows, I may choose to do things differently.

2. I feel guilty if I take time out to rest. I am not achieving enough.

2. It is good to take time out to rest when I feel tired. I can learn to maintain a good balance between doing and being. Being peaceful may be a greater achievement than anything else. Resting helps me feel my true self and be more energized.

JEALOUSY

1. I hate myself when I feel jealous of others and try to hide it.

1. Jealousy is only a lack of self love. I can learn to connect to my true self and be fed with love. The more I feel this love within myself, the more confident I am in my ability to learn and grow. Whatever is good for me will come to me. I can release myself from all comparisons.

2. I am afraid of feeling embarrassment or jealousy and must hide it from myself and others.

2. These are just sensations like any other sensations. The more authentic I am, the easier it is for me to feel all my feelings without judging them. I love all my feelings just as they are, including embarrassment and jealousy.

ANGER

1. I must get angry if someone hurts me or abuses me.

1. I can feel my anger momentarily and use that energy to focus on achieving my goals. No one can abuse me with their words if I don't abuse myself with toxic thoughts. I can choose to allow my

love to continue to flow and take care of myself appropriately.

RESENTMENT

1. I have to resent those who hurt me and seek revenge even though these feelings are poisoning me.

1. I can feel resentment momentarily and then convert it to love that helps heal me. The law of cause and effect will take care of them for hurting me. I don't have to make myself feel bad on top of it. I can choose to stop hurting myself further. It may be a lesson for me to learn from. I might have hurt someone else in a similar way and not be aware of it. One of the ways I learn is to experience what I did to others by others doing it to me. I then become more sensitive and aware of what it feels like and I stop hurting others.

2. When others hurt me, I want them to suffer.

2. When I sincerely pray and wish for others to feel good and have joyful, fulfilled lives, it makes me feel good inside. I am the one who benefits the most. When others feel good, they have no need to hurt me. Praying for my enemies is healing for me, and my body benefits by gaining more strength and health.

DOUBTING THE UNIVERSE

1. How can the universe give me disease and love me?

1. The universe is neutral. My body is giving me feedback, which will

help me grow mentally, emotionally, and spiritually. Disease gives me an evolutionary push to grow to be my true self. It is a message of love to create a more loving and fulfilling life.

2. How can there be so much suffering in the world if God loves us?

2. God or the universe can be likened to grandparents who love their grandchildren more than they love themselves. Sometimes the grandchildren have to experience pain in order to grow.

3. If I trust the universe, I may be wrong and end up disappointed.

3. Trusting is a good feeling that produces health. The more I trust myself, the more in alignment I am with the universe, and the more my trust in the universe grows.

4. I must always be in control. Being out of control is frightening and terrible.

4. When I let go of control and trust the universe, I gain authentic selfless control, and I function better.

Resources
Directory

DR. GOODMAN'S PROGRAM:
**Dr. Goodman's Healing and Prevention Support
Program for Individuals, Patients, Loved Ones,
Caregivers, and Healthcare Professionals**
This system gives you in-depth guidance on how to continue
your growth with the support of a powerful healing environment.
This program can be obtained at *www.youheal.com.*

DR. GOODMAN'S VIDEOS:
Self Healing and Pain Relief
60-minute video: $49.99.

**Empowerment and Prevention—
Self Healing Cancer** 60-minute video: $49.99.

**You Can Deserve the Best—
Journey to the Himalayas to Babaji's Center**
(includes 20-minute footage of Babaji filmed by David Berry)
60-minute video: $49.99.

Shipping and handling for videos,
$7 plus $3 for each additional item.

DR. GOODMAN'S AUDIOTAPES AND COMPACT DISCS:
Healing and Strengthening the Immune System
90-minute cassette tape: $19.99.

Teaching the Body to Heal Itself
40-minute cassette tape with music: $19.99.

**The Daily Healing Routine—
The 5-Minute, Three Times a Day Cure**
50-minute CD: $19.99, or cassette tape: $19.99.

Freedom from Pain, Anxiety, or Stress
50-minute CD: $19.99, or cassette tape: $19.99.
Shipping and handling for tapes or CDs,
$5 plus $2 for each additional item.

DR. GOODMAN'S BOOK:
Lessons from the Master:
One Woman's Journey to Self-Healing
149 pages: $19.99, plus $5 shipping and handling.
To order, send a check or money order to:
Dr. S. Goodman,
280 Hauoli St., Suite A17
Wailuku, Hawaii 96793, USA
E-mail: shdemag@aol.com. Website: *www.youheal.com.*

DR. O. CARL SIMONTON'S BOOK AND TAPES:
Getting Well—audiotapes
Getting Well Again—book
Simonton Cancer Center
P.O. Box 890
Pacific Palisades, CA 90272
800-338-2360. Website: *www.simontoncenter.com.*

MASTER MANTAK CHIA'S BOOK AND VIDEO:
The Inner Smile—book
Microcosmic Orbit—video
Healing Tao Foundation, 800-497-1017.

PAIN MANAGEMENT:

LOUISE L. HAY'S BOOKS:
You Can Heal Your Life and Heal Your Body
Website: *www.louisehay.com.*

DOLORES KRIEGER'S BOOK:
Accepting Your Power to Heal:
The Personal Practice of Therapeutic Touch
Website: *www.thehealingtouch.org.*

Ask Your Questions and Share Your Success Stories

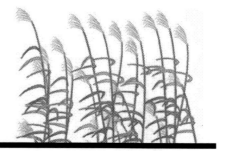

Shivani Goodman would like to hear your success stories and any feedback from family, friends, or clients. If you have questions about The 9 Steps Program, she will answer them in forthcoming books that will deepen the benefits of this book. To ensure confidentiality, your name, city, and state will be changed. Please send your questions and experiences to:

Dr. Shivani Goodman

280 Hauoli St., A-17, Wailuku

Hawaii, 96793, USA

Fax: 808-986-0505

Website: *www.youheal.com* Email: shdemag@aol.com.

Training Programs for Professionals and the Public

Dr. Goodman offers training programs for healthcare professionals and the public. Lectures; workshops; one-day, two-day and seven-day training sessions may be available in your area. For information about speaking engagements, workshops, and training programs, visit her Website at *www.youheal.com*. If you would like to invite Dr. Goodman to give a presentation to your group, contact her directly.

Supporting Instructors to Teach Worldwide

With the intention of erasing sickness, pain, and suffering, and fostering more joy, love, and peace in the world, a portion of the proceeds from this book will go toward training instructors to teach this program worldwide, particularly in poverty-stricken countries. If you wish to become an instructor or would like to contribute financially to help sponsor an instructor to teach in a particular city, state, or country, please contact Dr. Goodman. Your contributions are welcome and are appreciated.

Index

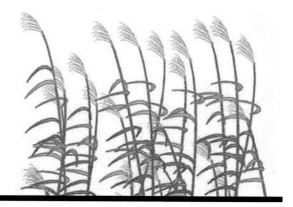

Index

Index